Life, Loss and Love

A Memoir By
Susan Nicholson

Edited by Sally Odgers and Meredith Swift

Cover Design by german_creative@fiverr

Formatted by Jen Henderson @Wild Words Formatting

Dedication

To my beloved mother (Moya Eva) who never left me and didn't forsake me when I was in such intense pain and sorrow. I will always love you so deeply and cherish you.

To my beloved sons Christopher and Matthew, and my precious grandchildren Behati, Leo and Chelsea. You all light up my life!

Train up a child in the way he should go,
and when he is old he will not depart from it.
Proverbs 22:6 (NKJV)

Table of Contents

Chapter 1

Beginnings

I came into the world on January 29, 1957, at the Queanbeyan Hospital. Queanbeyan NSW was known then as Struggle Town. This was an accurate description of my parents' situation as my mum and dad, Moya Eva Winch and Donald Nicholson, were very poor. For a time, they shared a home with Dad's parents, my uncles, Harry and Frank and my elder sister Maree, who was six-and-a-half years older than me.

When I was born, my mother had severe post-natal depression. She had to leave me for two weeks to recover, but I don't believe she ever fully did. At that time, my parents were living in their own flat in another part of Queanbeyan. My father and my aunties took over caring for me, bottle feeding me and making sure I was looked after properly. Mum had only two dresses—one she wore and one she washed. When she needed false teeth, the only way my father, who was a competitive bike rider, could afford to pay for them was to sell his bike.

For the first ten years of their marriage, my parents were very happy together. My mother was the third youngest of eight girls from a very strict Catholic family and all her sisters attended Catholic schools. My father, the youngest of three boys, came from a strict Anglican family. My father was so staunch in his Anglican faith that this was the religion I was raised in. I have my father to thank for taking me to church and instilling an awareness of God within me. He insisted that I attend confirmation and he took me to the midnight service on Christmas Eve.

Mum would never come to church with us, but her contribution was to make sure I was dressed beautifully, and she took a great deal of pride in this. I attended scripture lessons at school but took none of it seriously—rather, I saw this as a time to have fun!

When I was two, my parents moved into their own government home in the Canberra suburb of Forrest. A big flood came through that home not long afterwards and I remember being lifted into a manhole for safety. This very scary experience was my first childhood memory. Our car was washed away and, as a little child, this was very traumatic for me.

After the flood, the government gave my parents an option of another government home and my parents chose a house at 64 Dooring Street, Dickson. This new neighbourhood and home were the beginning of all my childhood memories; mostly good, but of course some sad times as well.

I spent all my childhood there. I was an active and outgoing little girl, who used to play outside a lot. I always had a dog in my life, which gave me a lot of comfort and kept me company. I got my love for animals, especially dogs, from my father. Neither my mother nor my sister had any time for them, and my sister never liked them near her. I had many dogs as a child but because we lived on a busy road, I lost almost all of them to cars. It was very distressing dealing with the loss of so many beautiful dogs. Especially traumatic for me was when my beloved dog Simon was thrown over our gates in one of my father's drunken episodes. I never saw Simon again and have no idea what became of him. I kept thinking of him and I coped by believing he found another home.

As well as my love for dogs, I adored dolls and was like a little mother to them all, playing with them for hours on end. I had a vivid imagination and would go into my own world. I had a name for each of my dolls and, to this day, I still remember these. My mother was very generous and I was always delighted at Christmas time or my birthday to get the latest and the best doll. I had a beautiful collection of them, and, as far as I was concerned, they were all real people. My sister wasn't into dolls at all and was happy with a beloved teddy bear named Moss. I think my mother delighted in having such an extroverted, high-spirited and excitable little daughter as me. I was a born leader—a little bit like the Pied Piper—with all the neighbourhood children following me. I created a group called the Tadpole Club and all the kids in the neighbourhood joined us.

I loved to organise activities and outings for the children in the Tadpole Club. On one occasion, we went up to the local fire station and got to go on the fire engine. On another, I organised a tour of the local ABC Radio Station. It was in my nature to be generous and giving and I loved to organise things which would make others happy. I organised meetings, plays and musicals for the residents of the nearby Goodwin Nursing Home. I used to make a booking for our performances and then take the Tadpole Club up to entertain the old folk. I also raised money for the Barnardos Homes for Children by selling cakes baked by my mother and aunties.

I was only young and would be so happy and excited to walk for a couple of miles to deliver $9 for children who were with Barnardos and didn't have a home of their own.

I loved playing with the other children and being out and about but there was a deeper reason as to why I was rarely inside my home. There was always an undercurrent of distress from my mother's anxiety and she simply could not cope with any of my friends coming over to play. We were never allowed to sit on our bedspreads or play inside. Mum would be drinking cups of tea and coffee with her friend Margaret and my auntie. To ensure that she wouldn't be disturbed, Mum sometimes switched on the electric floor cleaner and turned it upside down, still going, at the back door. It frightened me so much I never wanted to come inside while the floor cleaner was on. I remember my mother and whoever she was with at these times laughing because it was keeping us outside.

Mum did show her caring in other ways though. She made delicious home-cooked meals, our home was clean, I always had beautiful clothes and, compared to so many of my school friends, I felt privileged.

I attended North Ainslie Primary School. I remember feeling nervous in my first year there. My sister Maree and one of her friends were in sixth grade and came around only once to see me. They looked at me from the distance but didn't come to say "hello". I needed my sister to show she cared for me and I felt lonely and disappointed when she didn't.

Apart from the first day, when my mother dinked me on her bike, I walked all the way to school and back. This was not easy. I was only five years old, the walk was long, and I was frightened. Our North Ainslie uniforms were grey, and this made me easily identifiable as a public-school child. In contrast, the St Brigid's Catholic school uniforms were maroon. I was a clear target for bullying by these children; teased mercilessly and told I was going straight to hell. I would be so stressed and anxious that I would take little dolly steps, placing one foot in front of the other with no gap—heel to toes each step of the way. I lived in dread of what these Catholic school children would say and do to me.

I was relieved when I made a friend—a young boy—who walked the same route as me but on the opposite side of the road. We stayed friends throughout our childhood and when we were thirteen, he asked me to go steady with him. He was very kind, and his parents were beautiful to me, but I broke it off after six months as the relationship was too serious for where I was emotionally.

Another memory I have of my school days is of the milk we were given to drink. In those days, the government funded a milk program and every school child was given a free bottle of milk. Unfortunately, by the time we came to drink the milk, it would be warm from being in the sun. The taste of this warm milk made me want to vomit so Mum wrote a note to excuse me from having to drink it.

In the mornings, Maree and I would tiptoe around getting ready for school, in the hope our mother wouldn't wake up. If she did, it was like a nightmare, because she would be very angry. I remember my mother doing my hair in pony tails and she was pulling hard and hurting me. Maree said she could hear me screaming as she walked to the bus stop. I wished Maree would turn back and intervene; that she would defend me by saying something to our mother for this rough treatment. She never did.

Maree didn't have a strong, determined nature like mine. She was quieter and more compliant. I remember Maree was very frightened of needles of any sort and, to save her the distress, I found myself jumping in front of her for our annual flu injection. As a young child, she had also been very ill with hepatitis and for three months, Maree lay in her bed recovering. During that time, I would sit outside her bedroom door, chatting, telling jokes to make her laugh and ensuring she was not lonely. I think she loved me entertaining her with my non-stop happy chatting away, but she must have needed a break from my babbling! Even though we were very different in our natures, we really loved each other very much.

Before I came along, my sister was highly favoured and the centre of attention for the six-and-a-half years she lived with our grandparents. I had not lived with them the way Maree had, and they didn't know me very well. We had no real relationship and I didn't enjoy going to visit them as I felt ignored or misjudged, especially by my grandmother, Gwen. She would tell my parents, "You've got that child ruined!"

I think this was because she didn't understand my extroverted, determined and strong-willed personality. I was so different from my quieter and compliant elder sister. I remember when there was a leg of lamb bone in my grandparents' meat keeper and my grandmother told me, "And this is only for your sister." Things like this made it painfully obvious that Maree was her favourite.

It was a different story with my father's father, Jack, whom I called Pop. He was kind and gentle with me. Pop was the only grandparent I really loved and cared for. He always called me Lily. As an adult, I found out he called me this because Lily was the Hebrew meaning of Susan. I was always called Susie by the rest of my family.

My grandparents on my mother's side were not nice to me either. My mother's mother, Linda, was called Nanny and, when I was a little girl, I remember her being angry at me because I had used too much toilet paper. She passed away when I was about ten years old and I can only recall that one memory of her. Everyone in my family told me she was a lovely, kind lady but I didn't feel that way about her at all! And my mother's father Leo was scary! He would sit in the lounge room playing Ludo with my cousin Linda. She could stay inside with him while my other cousins Kathy and Peter played with me outside in their orchards. I have so many happy memories of this fabulous time with them. We stayed outside together for hours and hours. I think that kept my grandparents very happy and relaxed because they didn't have to deal with us. Because there was no real relationship with them, and no nice memories, it didn't bother me that I spent next to no time with them.

As I grew older, my mum went back to work packing bags at Coles supermarket. This meant Mum would not be there when I got home from school. I would see her stockings lying in the corner of the room and it made me miss her and feel anxious that something might happen to her.

One of Mum's often repeated sayings was, "You'll be sorry when I'm dead and gone." so when she was absent, I would suffer panic attacks and anxiety as I wondered whether she was still alive.

I did, however, enjoy having the house to myself. I would cook lamb chops under the griller and watch my favourite TV shows. Maree was a bit of a problem for me though. My growing up memories are very vague of my sister, probably because there was such a big age gap. Maree had started having boyfriends and would bring them home. I got sick of seeing her kissing her boyfriend and so, in order to make them stop, I took drastic measures. Brandishing a big knife, I forced them out of the house. This stopped their behaviour! My terrified sister reported back to Mum about what I had done, saying I was crazy and that I was going to kill them! Even though I was much younger, Maree was petrified of me.

I also remember dealing with my father going off his head when Maree was dating different boys. While she sat outside in her boyfriend's car canoodling with him, I would try to protect her by switching the outside light on and off, to let her know she had better get inside urgently before Dad went over the edge. My father was very distressed when Maree was dating a Catholic boyfriend and used to say, "No daughter of mine will be marrying a Catholic!" As far as my father was concerned, no boyfriend my sister brought home would ever be good enough.

Chapter 2
Growing Up

Time was passing, and Mum was eventually able to give up work at Coles. This was because my dad had become a very successful builder. He did not just build houses; he built whole suburbs. Dad's office was our dining room, where he would entertain clients. Our family went from being on the poverty line to becoming wealthy and privileged. My parents were able to afford very generous gifts for Christmas and birthdays. We were also able to go on extended family holidays in New South Wales and our favourite places were Kiama, Batemans Bay and Narooma. At the beginning of the first month, Dad would tow the caravan and set it up with our annexe at our holiday destination, and then he'd return for us, towing our boat. We would spend a month there and then Dad would return home to work while my sister, my mother and I would stay for another month.

Fishing was one of the things we enjoyed very much as a family. I remember being at Batemans Bay and drifting slowly along under the Clyde River bridge. Over the course of a few hours, I ended up catching twelve flathead. I was so excited! Mum enjoyed fishing with us but generally she found it hard to relax. She would be in the laundry talking to other women or cleaning up, with little time spent with Maree and me. I missed my mother and wished she was like my friends' mothers who spent quality time with them. Despite this, I was close to her and I would have to call myself a real Mummy's girl!

I think that came from the fact that my mother didn't show any favouritism. Even though my father sought out lots of quality time with both of us, he, like his mother, clearly favoured my sister.

Dad was only nineteen years old when he became a father and he used to call Maree "little sister", probably because she felt like a sister to him. He was kind and fun-loving, as well as being generous. He would pay for us to go to the local carnival where we would ride the popular Octopus or the Cha-Cha. I had no fear of the quick whizzing motion of these rides as we zig-zagged in and around. It was just pure fun for me! With my active, high-spirited and outgoing nature, I thoroughly enjoyed these wonderful family holidays. Some of my happiest childhood memories are of those times.

Sadly, there were other not so happy memories also being made. My parents' strong marriage had begun to weaken around the time my father's building career boomed. Dad had joined the Ainslie Football Club which was close to our home in Dickson. In those days, it was like a little shed and after a hard day's work building, he and his workmates would go there to unwind with a drink.

My mother was very anxious about my father's drinking. It became a pattern that, if my father came home at one minute to six, the mood in the house would be very good. On the other hand, if he arrived even one minute after six then it felt as though all hell had broken loose as my mother subjected him to a tirade of emotional abuse. When Mum was like this, Dad couldn't stay home, and he would return to the Football Club for another bellyful of alcohol.

This became a vicious cycle. The happy times of my parents' marriage had now given way to abuse and accusations. They were constantly fighting, and Maree and I would be caught in the middle, trying to appease Mum and stop her dreadful verbal abuse of Dad. We would literally beg her to leave our father alone. The constant stress and anger and the inevitable abuse of alcohol fuelled this destructive cycle. It would be late at night and my father in his drunken state would lament, "Nobody loves me, and nobody cares."

My sister and I would cry out in anguished reply, saying, "We do! We do!"

My father was also stressed by the big team of builders he had to manage. He developed a stutter and, when I was twelve, he had to be admitted to the Psychiatric Ward for treatment. While Dad was away, it was my responsibility to care for his large collection of tropical fish. For the whole month Dad was hospitalised, I carefully tended these fish and I was very proud that I never lost one of these temperamental creatures.

Dad was discharged, and life continued, with his business continually expanding. When I was fourteen, my parents announced they had bought land in Cook, A.C.T., and would be building a home there. They hadn't consulted me about this major decision, and I felt horrified and traumatised that I would have to leave the neighbourhood where I had grown up. It was the only neighbourhood I'd ever known, and I felt safe and secure there.

When we moved into our new home at Cook, I took my little chihuahua, Minnie, with us. Of all the many dogs I have owned, she was the dog I adored most of all, yet a tragic event almost ended Minnie's life when my mother and I were out in the front garden.

Suddenly, a black Labrador appeared. It pounced on Minnie, took her in its mouth and tossed her about like a rag doll. It took a superhuman effort from Mum and me to free Minnie. She was in very bad shape—barely moving and close to death—and it was imperative that we get her to a vet. Because my mother couldn't drive, we called for a taxi. Initially, the driver refused to take the three of us in his car, until my screams of hysteria made him change his mind. He finally gave in to our dire need for a taxi and we were able to get my beloved Minnie to the vet.

After examining Minnie, the vet told us that if a human can live with one lung then he could see no reason why a dog couldn't! He successfully operated on my beautiful Minnie and brought her back to health. Even though the vet bill came to $3,000—a lot of money in those days—Dad generously covered all costs. He knew how much I loved Minnie and how distressed and traumatised I was from what had happened to her. I remained so traumatised that I could never walk a dog again. Nor could I have two dogs close together, especially if they didn't know each other. Safely back at our new home in Cook, I lovingly nursed my strong and brave little dog back to full health.

The home at Cook was not just a simple house. It was a grand big home with all the latest features including an in-ground swimming pool. It was the early 1970s and this home seemed like a mansion to me. I felt such embarrassment because I was so used to being with children who had nothing and so I never invited anyone from school to visit me there. Unable to cope with the change, I would catch two buses from Cook to the city and then to Dickson High School in order to be back with my old school friends. Mum and Dad kept our house at Dickson, building a self-contained flat on the end of it. They rented this out while we lived at the new home in Cook.

Two years later, when I was sixteen, it was my parents who were in for a shock when I announced that I'd booked myself into the Metropolitan Business College and would not be returning to school. I had not consulted my parents about this, and they were understandably horrified. Maree had gone to the same Business College and was a stenographer, but I was determined I would not be learning shorthand. Being a secretary in an office would be far too boring for me. Because I loved being around people, I wanted to be a receptionist. I would need typing skills to help me gain the reception jobs I felt suited for.

Being a receptionist was what you might call my practical ambition. In addition, I had my heart set on becoming an actress. I used to imagine myself in all the dramas I watched on television. I had a vivid imagination and was in a few plays with leading roles but my parents weren't interested in coming to watch me perform. Because I was never encouraged in my acting ambitions, I settled for a steadier job, in which I worked around people in an encouraging and caring role, so I wanted to learn typing and get out of Business College as quickly as possible. I was starting to make decisions for what was best for me, and to take responsibility for what I wanted in my life. I was growing up.

Chapter 3

Trust and Betrayal

I was growing up and spreading my wings, and this extended to my growing awareness of the opposite sex. Over the course of my young life, I had already started to develop feelings for boys. During one of our holidays in Kiama, my mother had befriended a family from Sydney, with whom we eventually became very close. One of their sons was near Maree's age and another one was only a couple of years older than me.

At the tender age of seven, this boy became my first crush. We stayed in contact with the family, and when Maree got married, she invited them to the wedding. By then I was fourteen, and this boy, who was sixteen, began writing to me in Canberra from his home in Sydney.

After I finished Business College, Dad decided I would move to Sydney. He arranged for me to board with some friends of his who had four children. One of their children was a little deaf and dumb boy. I didn't know this family very well, but I was often expected to mind the four children on my own. This was difficult for me, as I had no experience in this area. I also felt quite lonely and I had only my boyfriend for comfort. He was just beautiful to me, but he was studying for his HSC and his mother was concerned about his studies. He wasn't allowed to see me much. Even though the family knew me well, I guess I was a distraction for him.

Things were made easier by my father's regular visits to Sydney. These visits enabled Dad to buy tropical fish to add to his large collection. It was Dad who was responsible for me securing my first job, as a dental nurse and receptionist in Croydon. I had to catch public transport from where I boarded in Homebush. Once I ended up on the wrong train to Redfern, which back then was one of the less reputable parts of Sydney. Often, I would be on a train home when it was dark. I would have to walk across a park to get to where I was boarding and this was quite daunting.

I was homesick, and this was made worse by the fact that I never heard from my mother for the six months I was in Sydney.

I think minding four children, living in a home that was not kept up to the standards I was used to, and not having any friends, all combined to make me want to go back to Canberra. After six months, I decided to quit my job and return home. My father didn't take this well at all and he was very angry, abusive and threatening towards me. He kept saying he had set me up and got me a job and he didn't want me to leave. Despite this, I stuck to my decision.

I was shocked when I learned the real reason my father had been visiting Sydney. It turned out that he was having an affair with the wife of the family I was living with! When I found out about this, I felt both betrayed and exploited. Because he visited me so much in Sydney, I had thought he cared about me. I was devastated to find out this was just an excuse to conduct an affair.

It had been left to me to look after the four children, so my father could go out partying with their parents. This was a very strict Catholic family, and the wife ended up having a breakdown over the affair.

I felt caught up in the middle of all of this, with no idea as to what had been going on. Upon my return home, I was in for another huge shock. My father was living in the bigger family home in Cook and my mother was back in our ex-government home in Dickson. The reason she hadn't contacted me was because she'd met up with an old boyfriend and was now living with him. They had first met when my mother was fourteen and then they lost touch for many decades. They reconnected again when he was a barman at the Hotel Queanbeyan which my mother had chosen as the venue for my sister's wedding reception. It was then that the affair began.

Returning to Canberra and to the reality of my parents' divorce after twenty-three years of marriage was devastating. I was only sixteen, it was Christmas Eve, and I had to make a snap decision as to whether I should live with my mother or my father. I chose my mother. I had been so homesick and wondering why she hadn't contacted me during my time in Sydney. Even though I loved her and wanted to be with her, I also lost respect for her because she was living with a man who was not my father.

The same night I chose to live with my mother, she and her boyfriend went out. I have never felt so lonely and lost as on that Christmas Eve, all alone after returning from living in Sydney. Mum was so proud of herself, all beautifully dressed and adorned with jewellery. Later, I could hear the sounds through my bedroom wall when they made love. I put a pillow over my ears to block out the noise.

To make matters worse, Maree's marriage had broken down. She had not been married long and had an eighteen-month-old son, Andrew.

I was still at high school when Maree had fallen pregnant with Andrew and I was one of the first people she confided in. Maree was very excited about the prospect of becoming a mother, but I was worried sick about my father's reaction, especially as she wasn't married or engaged, and the father of her baby was from a strict Catholic family. I would pace the floor until well after midnight and my mother was very concerned about my behaviour! When Maree finally told my parents the news about her pregnancy, my father's reaction was one of rage and disbelief. He had her so high up on a pedestal and he was unable to accept that Maree could ever do anything wrong. It was up to me and one of Maree's friends to try to convince him that Maree was telling him the truth.

Lashing out at me, my father said he would have expected an unplanned pregnancy from me and that he would be locking me away in the bathroom. I was very distressed by his reaction and felt it was typical of the way he always compared his compliant child (Maree) with his high-spirited child (me). My father always said the mould was broken when Maree was born, and this sort of comment went on all our lives. I was also distressed because I was still a virgin and so I felt unfairly judged and condemned by my father.

The next day I came home to find my little chihuahua Minnie was gone. We couldn't find her anywhere! My mother eventually found out my father had taken her down to the local vet to be de-sexed. This was my father's way of coping with Maree's sudden and unexpected announcement. Honestly, so much of my childhood was a complete circus! I think I made a subconscious decision I would never be the type of parent my mother was, and I would never marry someone like my father. Despite this, I still really loved both of my parents.

After my return from Sydney, I was at my lowest ebb. I responded to what was happening by being very rebellious, especially to my mother as she had lost my trust and respect. In order to cope with the emotions, stress and confusion I was experiencing during this time of turmoil, I tried group counselling. I felt so very lost and alone.

Even though I was emotionally devastated, I knew I needed to find a job. I applied for and was accepted as a dental nurse and receptionist in Kingston. The dentist, a Greek man named George, did not take on girls under nineteen for reception. However, I was able to persuade him to give me a trial for three months, to prove to him that I was able to do the job.

I needed to catch two buses to get to my job, but it was within walking distance of where one of my aunties lived. At lunchtime, I would visit her, and she would serve up a beautifully cooked meal. I was still in contact with my boyfriend in Sydney who, without fail, would ring me at my auntie's place. I loved my boyfriend so much and looked forward with great excitement to his call.

Amidst this time of turmoil, he was a rock of stability, but Sydney felt so far away from me. And now, with my parents divorced, my perception towards my boyfriend was changing. I believed he was too good-looking to be interested in me and his mother didn't encourage our relationship. That made me feel I wasn't good enough for him or for his family. His parents were still together, and I now came from a broken home. My self-esteem and self-worth were at rock bottom.

Even though I was very committed and sincere in my long-distance relationship I was lonely and feeling very lost. I was catching up with old friends I had missed while living in Sydney and I found myself attracted to another guy. I was waiting at the bus stop when he stopped and said he needed to get something from the railway station. This was close to where I worked in Kingston and so he offered me a lift to work. There I was, dressed in my dental nurse uniform of a white mini-skirt and patent leather flat shoes, accepting his offer at face value. It wasn't just a lift he was after! This was his way of asking me to go steady.

I felt so broken and lonely from the painful changes in my life and the grief and heartbreak that my parents were no longer together. My boyfriend felt a million miles away. I couldn't explain what was happening to me and at only sixteen, I didn't have the emotional maturity to deal with it all. Besides, in the 1970s things like this were just not discussed. I felt torn—caught in the crossfire of my boyfriend ringing me every day and another nice and fun-loving guy wanting to go steady with me. In the 70s, guys who liked you asked if they could go steady and bought you a friendship ring. It was so innocent back then compared to today with all the online dating.

My boyfriend drove down from Sydney and I was embarrassed and confused. not feeling able to tell him the real reason—which was that I didn't feel good enough for him. I kept wondering why he would be interested in me. By that stage, he was working in a bank and I figured he could get anyone he wanted. I ended up breaking up with him and then I started dating the new guy in Canberra.

My new boyfriend was the second of six children and his mum was just beautiful to me. This was a welcome change from the disapproval I had felt from my previous boyfriend's mother. I experienced a great deal of freedom within my new relationship. I think it was better for me because my boyfriend and I both lived in the same city and I wasn't feeling so lost and lonely. There was also a sense of understanding in my new relationship because my boyfriend's parents were breaking up and I felt this made us even. It's sad to think that at the tender age of sixteen I was so insecure and had such low self-worth. I put this down to living in a dysfunctional alcoholic family.

I was still living with my mother and her new boyfriend and, because she was so busy with him, she didn't seem to care where I was or what time I came in. I was spending lots of time with my new boyfriend and enjoying my job as a receptionist/dental nurse for George. Even though I loved my job and I was very happy working for George, I was soon presented with an opportunity to switch careers and go nursing. So, at the age of seventeen, I moved into the Nurses' Quarters, sharing with lots of other girls, mostly from the country.

This was my second time living out of home and it was a very different experience for me. There was a lot of smoking—both cigarettes and marijuana—among the girls. I never touched either of these, but I would often finish my shift and find the girl rostered on for the next shift was too stoned to wake up. There was constant partying and many of the girls slept around. I was not used to this type of reckless behaviour and morally, it went against everything I stood for. On one occasion, I was humiliated when I was stripped naked and thrown in the shower. There would be girls hanging off the balconies in the Nurses' Quarters and the police were a constant presence. I found the whole scene distressing. I was out of my depth and I was not coping at all. Four months in, I decided to leave.

I couldn't bring myself to tell my parents the truth behind my decision. Instead, I told them I was too distressed by the number of people dying in the recovery area after surgery.

When George the dentist found out I had left nursing, he offered me my old job back. I decided against this and instead opted to be part of a typing pool with the Public Service in the Defence Department. In contrast to my dental nurse/reception job, I hated being in the typing pool. I was still going out with my boyfriend and I had fallen madly in love with him, but things were not smooth sailing with this relationship, and I ended up breaking up with him after two years of dating.

The problem was, he was friends with another couple, who had a little child. They were new to Canberra and my boyfriend wanted to spend a lot of time with them. I didn't feel particularly safe around this couple as it was obvious that the female was after him and the male was after me. I didn't want to be part of this relationship with them.

Things came to a head one night when my boyfriend picked me up and I agreed to go back to his place for dinner, cooked by his mother. I told him I would do this only on the condition that we didn't go back to this couple's place afterwards. My boyfriend agreed but then he changed his mind and wanted to go to their place after all. I demanded that he drop me back at my home and slammed the door in his face, telling him, "That's it! We're over and I'm never getting back together with you again!"

I was heartbroken, but I stayed true to my word and I never did get back with him. As had been the case with my previous boyfriend, I was unable to tell him the real reason for our breakup. It took a lot of courage and strength to stay broken up with him. He reminded me too much of my father and, because I had been so affected by Mum's accusations of Dad, I was afraid he wouldn't stay faithful to me.

I was totally devastated by the end of this relationship and it took me many years to recover.

I was invited to a family wedding by my previous boyfriend from Sydney. I spent a few days with him there. He was heading for a banking position and relocating to Darwin after it had been destroyed by Cyclone Tracy. I wanted to ask him to reconcile with me, but in the end, I didn't have the confidence to go through with this. I wanted to explain to him how I saw him as rock-solid and with excellent morals. I had loved him for so long—since I was a little girl of seven—and I still loved him very much. I saw him off at the airport when he was leaving for Darwin and he gave me a tender kiss goodbye. I was confused by what the kiss meant but once again, I didn't have the emotional maturity to express myself. I just couldn't find the words or confidence to talk to him about how I was feeling, and I let him go. I couldn't believe I let this opportunity pass me by, but I thought he was so good-looking and would meet someone nicer than me!

I was still with the Public Service working in the typing pool. Emotionally, I was at a very low ebb, but professionally I was doing well, being transferred to a better position within the Defence Department. It was there that I met Richard, my future husband. I was eighteen, and he was four years older. I was attracted to Richard because he was steady and stable—not a womaniser—and very kind and shy. These qualities appealed to me. We began dating, but I was still grieving the loss of my two-year relationship with my previous boyfriend and the fact that I couldn't talk to my Sydney ex-boyfriend, who now lived in Darwin.

After dating for a year, things were getting too serious with Richard. I wasn't comfortable with our relationship, and I wanted to run.

I had a close girlfriend, Kerri, and, despite having no money, we decided to go to New Zealand. To me, this was an opportunity to take some time out from my relationship with Richard and my broken heart over the lost love of my previous boyfriend. My father was worried that Kerri and I would be hitchhiking because a young Australian backpacker had recently been murdered in New Zealand. His last words to me were, "Don't hitchhike!" but that didn't stop me from doing just that. Kerri and I travelled around, backpacking and staying in youth hostels on the North Island. On the South Island the weather was much colder, so we didn't hitchhike much. We preferred the warmth of catching buses.

I really loved the travelling lifestyle. To pay my way, I found a job at *The Waterloo,* a pub in Wellington on the North Island. My next job was as a housemaid at a ski lodge in Queenstown on the South Island. These two jobs sustained me, and Kerri and I enjoyed our time away so much that we spoke of travelling to Europe when we returned.

I was looking forward to this and I was refreshed and excited when I came home to Canberra. My sister and her new boyfriend, Laurie, picked me up from the international airport. Richard was with them and he gave me a very expensive gift of a cassette player. I felt pressured and obligated to Richard for a gift that I felt was out of step with the level of my feelings for him. My mother was also putting pressure on me to be with Richard. Unknown to me, my ex-boyfriend from Sydney had been ringing my mother's home while I was in New Zealand, but she hadn't passed these messages on to me. Upon my return from New Zealand, Mum's first words to me were, "Don't you dare hurt that boy."

Richard was crying a lot and had some sort of breakdown while I was away because he couldn't cope without me. My mother was consoling him by cooking baked meals for him. His own mother, Dorothy, had let me know on several occasions that her son was not emotionally strong. I didn't quite know what this meant, probably because I was so independent and strong-willed, though lacking the emotional maturity and confidence to express my feelings. When Richard proposed to me, I told him I wasn't ready for the responsibility of marriage. I wanted to go travelling in Europe.

He wouldn't take no for an answer and his response was, "If you love me, you'll marry me, and you'll make this work."

I felt damaged and insecure by the failure of the marriages of the key people in my life—my parents and Maree. But more than this, I felt controlled by what my mother and Richard wanted and so I caved under the pressure and agreed to the marriage.

Five months later, on May 29, 1976, I was in my wedding gown in the car with my father on the way to the church.

My father asked, "Are you sure this is what you want, Sunny?" (This was his pet name for me.)

I nodded yes, but inside I was saying, "It's a bit late now."

Chapter 4
Marriage and Motherhood

At nineteen, I had become a married woman. Richard and I had a lovely honeymoon on Hayman Island. We came home to live in the self-contained flat adjoining our old family home in Dickson, paying rent at the going rate as Mum was not financially able to give it to us cheaply. Richard started to become very controlling with money and I couldn't even spend 10c on a chocolate Paddle Pop without him noticing the money was missing. Even though we had dated for over a year, this aspect of his character had not revealed itself to me.

As a new bride, I was cooking and cleaning and working full-time. I used to get very tired. Richard would work overtime, and I would go to pick him up. One night, feeling particularly exhausted, I fell asleep and woke at 9.00 pm. I went to pick Richard up and looked out for him on the side of the road as I drove to his workplace. He was a very good rugby league player and very fit and I thought he might be running home. It turned out that this was just what he'd done and when I got home, I found him in the shower. He refused to speak to me, and he ended up giving me the silent treatment.

I couldn't talk with Richard about the reason I failed to pick him up on time. This wasn't the first time we had been unable to communicate over deeper issues that affected us.

When I was eighteen and newly engaged, despite using contraception, I had fallen pregnant. There was no talk or consideration that we would keep the baby and I felt I had no choice but to have an abortion. Richard wouldn't tell me his reasons for not wanting the baby. Was it because he was the only son among three daughters and didn't want to let his parents down? Could it have been that I would have to give up work to have the baby and we couldn't afford the loss of income? I could only guess at the reason.

I went ahead with the abortion, which was performed at the Canberra Hospital, and, apart from severe cramping, I didn't feel much affected. I had no self-awareness and I had spent my whole life not being able to identify my feelings. Both my parents had put Richard up on a pedestal so much that I was at a point emotionally where I felt so lucky to have him. I believed everything he said was of great value. I didn't oppose him or dispute with him in any way. Later, though, the decision to go ahead with the abortion came back to haunt me and I felt deeply affected by the loss of this beautiful baby, who would now be forty-three. Not a day goes by where I don't think about the fact I could have a beautiful daughter or a third son now!

I was also experiencing pain and vomiting up bile and I had seven major attacks of pain that put me on the floor after eating certain foods. I was unwell off and on for twelve months and I finally found out I had gallstones. In those days there were no ultrasounds or keyhole surgery, so I had to undergo major surgery to have my gallbladder removed. As a young bride, I found it very traumatic trying to get a diagnosis and then having to go through major surgery. Richard was very supportive and good to me through this process.

Now that we were married, Richard and I planned to start a family. Before this could happen, we wanted to have a home of our own. I asked my dad if he would build me a house and he agreed to do so only if we could pay cash for a block of land first. Within twenty months, we had saved $7500. There was a block of land we wanted to purchase, located at 1 Snowy Place, Kaleen.

My father was drinking heavily and had plenty of women young enough to be my sister. He didn't want to go through with building a house for us, being against the idea and calling it a "love job". He wanted us to wait for land in a different suburb, but this was just an excuse not to build for us. My mother was very upset that my father refused to honour his promise to us. She was the one who would back me up and go into bat for me. I could always rely on this part of her nature.

In this case, Mum went above and beyond to find a builder for us and in the end, it was a distant cousin of hers, Viv Cooper, who got the job. Viv was a very good builder and he did an excellent job on our house. To save money, Richard and I would do all the labouring on the building site at the end of the day. We would go there after work and clean up. We were very happy working together towards our common goal of a home of our own.

The building was not without its problems, however. Our block of land was positioned on a creek bed, and over half our house—three bedrooms, lounge, and dining room—was situated on landfill. We had to pour nine feet of concrete at a cost of $700. After having to pay extra for the concrete, we could not afford to buy the fan-forced oven we wanted. We chose to miss out on the oven so our home could be completed.

On February 12, 1978, Richard and I moved from our little flat into our lovely new three-bedroom home with one bathroom, one toilet, family room, a lounge and dining room. We felt as though we were living in the lap of luxury! We were very excited and happy. We got on well together and, as time went on, I grew to really love and respect Richard. I was a good homemaker, cooking and cleaning capably. My mother and everyone who knew me couldn't believe how organised and thorough I was in every detail of our lives. I would have to say that I was very much an idealist and I loved being a homemaker.

Living in our beautiful new home and with life running smoothly, it was time for us to start our family. I was now twenty-two. Richard and I were very keen to purchase a good reliable family car before I became pregnant. We saved enough money to buy a brand new Holden Commodore, the first one to hit the market. But at the last minute I found myself having to pick up our new car by myself when Richard said he had a headache. I was capable and strong and took this in my stride, listening to the instructions from the Holden dealer on all the modern features of this beautiful new car. I was driving it home and everyone was looking at the car because it was the latest model.

It should have been such an exciting time, but I couldn't help feeling alone with this excitement. Looking back on that time and finding Richard with his headache, I now realise that his inability to cope with change or any major event was a pattern of his personality. I remember that this was also evident when Richard got one of his friends to do the photography for our wedding. Most of the photos didn't turn out, and those that did were of bad quality. I was so devastated, but I saw a solution. We could get dressed up again, as we still had the bridesmaids' dresses and the wedding dress, and we only needed to hire the suits again. But once again, due to Richard's inability to cope with change, I received another definite no—and more disappointment.

I fell pregnant and our son was born on December 28, 1979. We named him Christopher because he was born at Christmas time and his name means Christ bearer. I had no real sense of God, even though I had been raised and married in the Anglican faith. My pregnancy with Chris didn't go well and six weeks before he was due, I went to have a check-up. My gynaecologist told me I had toxaemia and that I needed to be in hospital urgently. I was only twenty-two and on my own and so I started to cry. The gynaecologist calmed me down and had me go home and pack my bag. I was ordered to have complete bed rest in hospital. I wasn't even allowed up to go to the toilet so I had to use a bed pan in the bed.

After a week I was allowed home on one condition—that I had to lie with my head down for the rest of the pregnancy. I did everything I was told and made it to full-term and the gynaecologist decided to induce me a day earlier than the due date. This was a long and difficult labour. At 7.00 am I was induced, and I had an epidural for the last hour because my blood pressure was soaring, and Christopher's heartbeat was in distress. The gynaecologist was very concerned and decided to put my legs up in stirrups and performed a high forceps delivery at 8.40 pm that night.

Despite all this trauma, it was so exciting that I was giving birth! Chris came out with his eyes wide open and all this beautiful hair with blond tips. My father was so excited about it all that he said he was the father and somehow, he managed to get into the labour ward. We were all beside ourselves as we had not had a baby in my family since my nephew Andrew was born eight years earlier.

Chris was a very difficult baby. He was full of colic and feeding was very hard work and took me hours. I went to the Queen Elizabeth Home to get some help with the feeding problems Chris had. I was unable to breastfeed because I had undergone a breast reduction when I was eighteen. I had visited a plastic surgeon when I was seventeen and his advice was to go away and think about the reduction for a year before I made any final decision. I was very slight, only about forty kilos, but I was top heavy and way out of proportion. This was further emphasised by the fitted, stretchy fashion of the 1970s. There was no doubt in my mind that I desperately needed the reduction. I was grateful to have the full support of my mother in this. Because it was such a big reduction, the operation took a full three hours.

I put all of Christopher's problems with colic down to me not being able to breastfeed him. I was only twenty-two and despite all the crying and the colic, as well as the sleep deprivation, I coped well and took everything in my stride. However, it was a very different story for Richard, who as usual did not cope well with a major change. For example, when Chris was a newborn being helped with his feeding problems, Richard begged me to go to the Canberra Show with him rather than pick up our beautiful baby from the Queen Elizabeth Hospital. I found it quite amusing because Richard didn't even like the Canberra Show, but I think it was his last-ditch effort at having time away from a crying baby with colic. We didn't go to the show and took Christopher back home, which is what I really wanted to do.

Richard had just started a new job in a different department of the Public Service and the stress of this, coupled with a newborn baby in the house, led to him having a nervous breakdown. For a time, Richard was unable to work, or even look after the beautiful garden he'd been working on. Even with all these challenges, I just got on with things and did what needed to be done.

I had a conversation with Richard's boss in the Department of Transport, explaining the situation to him. As a result, things were adjusted and made easier for Richard and he was therefore able to cope much better. Once Richard was able to get some support in his new job, he was able to enjoy Chris and he became a fantastic father. He took lots of videos and photographs of Chris and was an excellent hands-on father in every sense.

Our home was comfortable and always clean and tidy. In the backyard we had a sandpit, a cubby house, slippery slide, trampoline and a little swimming pool. There was a barbeque area as well as a huge vegetable garden where Richard loved to grow fresh vegies. I was so happy to be able to stay at home in this lovely environment for Christopher's first twelve months of life.

Unfortunately, we were under pressure financially with two mortgages and it was expected that I would go back to work in the Public Service. I was in the Office of National Assessments, Prime Minister and Cabinet, having been promoted from Defence at the time I went on maternity leave. It was a high security area, working with economists who analysed Australia's relationships with other countries. I rang up the Director of the ONA and explained I would like to return to work, but only work when my sister could mind Christopher. I was delighted when he created a new position for me! I worked Monday and Friday and stayed in this position until I was seven months pregnant again.

Richard and I became parents again when our second son, Matthew, was born on September 8, 1982. At that stage, the night before Matthew was born was the only time in my life that I got down on my hands and knees and prayed to God to go into labour. Richard was working back late, and I had put Chris to bed. I was feeling very unwell and desperate with fatigue. I remember feeling very tired halfway through the pregnancy. I was having regular blood tests and ultrasounds because I had been having almost no movement from the baby. This was a totally different pregnancy to Chris's and not having your baby move much was a real concern!

I awoke the morning after I had prayed and I was in the early stages of labour, with Matthew being born at 1.00 pm. I never thought another thing about whether God answered that desperate prayer.

Richard had always believed he would have daughters and it was quite a shock for him to instead be the father of two sons! When I was asked what our newborn son's name was, I was delighted to say Matthew with two Ts which meant "Gift from God" in Hebrew. Richard and I had discussed names but he was in such shock at being the father of two sons that I was able to say "Matthew" with excitement and delight!

Matthew was born three weeks early and his birth was extremely distressing. He was another high forceps delivery because all my contractions just stopped, and they needed to get Matthew out quickly. He was born crying and crying, and I was in so much pain that I couldn't enjoy or take it all in for some time.

It was a Wednesday that Matthew came into the world. In the Canberra Hospital they had a policy that no visitors were allowed on Wednesdays in the Maternity section. The exception to this rule was when a new baby had been delivered. I was shocked when Richard didn't want any close family members coming up to meet Matthew as he was delivered at lunchtime. He told the family no visitors were allowed on a Wednesday and that night, when I was all fresh and ready to share my joy, none of our families came to meet our beautiful little Matthew. It was very hard for me when I couldn't have anyone to visit, but I was so naïve and hung off every word Richard said, unable to express my feelings of disappointment.

I was told when Matthew was born that he had been living in the littlest sac the doctors had ever seen! He was born with a torticollis tumour and his head only went to one side. It was very distressing because when I heard the word "tumour", I thought Matthew had cancer. There was a lot of physio involved and I was told he was either too cramped inside my womb or the high forceps delivery caused the torticollis tumour. We were advised Matthew should have an operation to correct his neck muscle when he was older, but we weighed up the pros and cons and decided against something so radical. Numerous times a day while he was asleep, I would move his head to stretch the muscle. I did this for many years and eventually it was corrected as best it could be.

Before Matthew was born and when Christopher was two, Richard's adored grandmother was in Melbourne visiting family and friends when she suddenly suffered a massive heart attack. Richard's childhood had been very hard and sad. His father was a gambler and an alcoholic and Richard was forever protecting his mother. He told me she wasn't well and at one stage he did all the housework. His grandmother had helped ease the pain of Richard's childhood and played a hugely important role in his life. He had always said she was the only one that gave him love! She was a beautiful Nanna and very excited and good to her great-grandchildren. I loved the way she cared for and treated Chris, and I can only imagine what an amazing grandmother she was to Richard.

We had just returned from a coastal holiday and Richard flew to Melbourne to be by her side in hospital. At this stage, we were all hoping she would pull through but sadly she passed away in Melbourne and her body was flown back to Canberra so we could arrange her funeral. I could never have been prepared for the radical change we as a family were about to undergo. The husband I farewelled at the airport was to return to me as a very different man.

Chapter 5

For the Love of My Sons

Richard's outlook on life had radically changed by the time he came home from Melbourne. It was as though he was a completely different man. He wanted to talk to me about God, but it was as though he was speaking a foreign language. I didn't have the faintest idea of what he was talking about.

Richard experienced a revelation of Jesus when he became a charismatic, born again Christian. He said God had revealed Himself to him while he was with his dying grandmother.

My sister Maree had a deep faith from four years of age, and she was so excited by Richard's conversion because she now had someone to share her faith journey with! Maree and Richard began to attend every Christian conference, meeting and service they could. Christian wall plaques and books began appearing in our home. My husband was rarely home, and when he was, it was as though he was a stranger to me. It was as though I had lost him to God—as well as to my sister. I found the whole experience very confronting and intimidating.

Richard did not want to give up on our marriage. The Bible had clear instructions about the importance of staying married and Richard was praying and praying for me to become a Christian. I decided I would stay with him and that we would attend church as a family, providing it was the Anglican church where I was married, and which was the familiar faith I had been raised in. Christopher attended Sunday School and when Matthew turned three, he was to join his big brother. The plan was that Richard was just going to settle Matthew into Sunday School and then he would come to the remainder of the church service with me.

Instead, Richard ended up staying for the whole of the Sunday School session and running a charismatic program for the children.

While Richard was very much alive in the Spirit, I was very much dead. I found the women of the Anglican church to be quite snobbish and not at all down to earth like the friends I was used to. I volunteered for everything I could think of, putting my name down to do flowers for weddings, serve on the church committee and help with canvassing for bequeaths. I found this very difficult as I was expected to visit old people in their nursing home who were parishioners of this Anglican church. I felt so intimidated and I was doing things I was not good at and which did not come naturally for me—for example, doing the flowers, of which I hated every minute.

For three years I stayed there, constantly on the roster and doing all that I could. I felt dead to the spiritual realm and I had no revelation of God at all.

Richard was on fire for the Lord, but the danger was that he was in the honeymoon phase of being a new Christian and was not being mentored at all. There was some dispute and he wanted to leave that church and soon he had found another Anglican church for us to join. I was very unhappy and didn't want to go to church full-stop but found myself in another church of Richard's choice just to please him!

Fortunately, the intimidation I felt around the Anglican church ladies was a small part of my life at that time. I was a stay-at-home mum and Snowy Place was, without a doubt, an ideal place to raise a young family. It was a cul-de-sac of seven houses and our neighbours were friendly, caring and supportive.

I was also part of a group of young mothers, who became the most wonderful social network and an amazing support for me. All of us had new babies and new homes in different suburbs near each other. We were all battling financially, with double mortgages, and we started with sheets up at our windows and made do with old furniture until we could afford to slowly replace it. We were all happy and excited for one another whenever anything was bought which added to the décor of our homes. I remember being so excited just to buy something as simple as a new kitchen bin! It was wonderful to see us all complete our family homes. We would all meet—with our young children—at each other's homes for morning tea or lunch. We would have "girls' nights" together at each other's homes while our husbands minded the children. We would drink wine and coffee, and eat delicious savoury food, followed by homemade slices and cakes.

Our husbands also got on well with each other so we would attend wonderful fancy dress/theme parties at neighbourhood homes while our young children were minded. All our friends adored Richard—as well as being a great sportsman, he was also a great dad. I used to give Richard two weeks' notice about any up and coming party or event. I found this approach worked best for him because it gave him plenty of time to get used to the idea that we were all going to dress up in our fancy dress outfits. He always joined in and he loved these years as much as I did. I remember for one fancy dress I decided to go as a nun. My neighbour Kath's sister was a nun, so I was able to borrow the whole outfit from her. I saw this as a bit of fun but when I look back, I find it hard to believe I asked to borrow a nun's habit! There I was, carrying a Bible in one hand and with a stubbie of beer in the other. Richard was totally against me drinking alcohol and would get very angry if I had a laugh and would blame it on the few wines, so I always knew to not get giggly. I didn't have an alcohol problem, but I respected and loved him so much that I did what he wanted. He was emotionally affected by his childhood and his father's drinking habits.

Once a year, my friends and I would have a full girls' weekend together and go away up to Sydney by train. We would watch a live musical production. This was such a special weekend and we would save for a whole year to be able to go! Richard and all the other husbands were supportive of this and they looked after the children. Because I didn't want Richard to be stressed about the financial side of things, I would try to save one-dollar coins for the whole year. These were the best years of my entire life and I will always be grateful for this wonderful social network. I was never lonely with these amazing women in my life!

Number 1 Snowy Place was like a central meeting place for all the neighbourhood children. Both Christopher and Matthew have amazing memories of their childhood. During school holidays there would be an array of neighbours and children the boys would play with from first thing in the morning until early in the evening, only stopping when it was time for dinner, bath and bed. Christopher and Matthew had lots of friends and everyone was welcome into our lovely home. I ran the house capably, with only a rare occasion that Richard would come home to the toys not being put away or the sandpit cover left off. If there was any disarray at all he could not cope, and I just had to wait for time to pass and everything was good again.

Richard and I worked well together to give both our sons the most amazing birthday parties. On one occasion, I hired a magician to add that touch of magic! I would cook all the children's cakes out of the *Women's Weekly* magazine. The boys would pick the one they liked, and I would create it for them. For the parents—mostly mothers—we had a big urn for tea and coffee in our shed as well as homemade cakes and slices. It was a hive of activity that was so much fun! To this day, both Chris and Matthew have lasting childhood memories of these wonderful, magical parties.

For Christmas lunch, Richard and I used to do the same for both sides of our families. I remember arranging our furniture and decorating the long trestle table and we had everyone sitting together. We moved our furniture into a gauzed outside room (called the green room) and after lunch we would all overflow between the rooms, relaxing and enjoying each other's company. We were blessed that both our families got along so well. Richard and I really enjoyed working together to organise these occasions, which were just wonderful! For an extended time before and after Christmas, Richard's grandfather would stay with us. He was a delight to have around and was very much treasured by the whole family, especially Chris and Matthew. They loved their great grandfather—who they called old Pop—so very much! Richard couldn't cope with anyone other than his grandfather staying with us at this time of year. He needed his peace and quiet and I respected this because I loved him.

Christopher was born three days after Christmas and I was determined that he would not miss out on a birthday celebration. This was probably because I was never given a party as my mother couldn't cope. No sooner had Richard and I cleaned up after the big Christmas family gatherings than we would be preparing for and going straight back into full swing for Chris's birthday—especially before he started school. When Chris was older and had school friends, we would often celebrate his birthday before school broke up for the Christmas holidays.

Both Richard and I loved our sons so much. He was a real "hands-on" father—capable and very practical. It was like working with another female as we complemented each other so well. I would have all the ideas and, even though it took Richard a while to come around, he usually did—especially where his beloved sons were concerned. He was a very good rugby league football player who often received trophies for Best and Fairest, as well as being Captain/Coach. While I was pregnant with Chris, Richard suffered a back injury that had the potential to cause paraplegia. Because of this, he was very opposed to his sons following in his footsteps and playing rugby league football. Instead, he encouraged them into soccer, and he was coach for Chris's team, while Matthew played in a younger age group. Richard and I were our sons' biggest fans and we loved supporting them!

Richard and I were both fully committed to nurturing our boys and developing their gifts. Even though I had no self-awareness as to my own nature, I was very cued into the different personalities of my boys and I was aware of what they both needed in order to flourish. There were similarities—Christopher and Matthew were both kind, caring, well-behaved and easy to manage.

Christopher's personality reminded me very much of myself with the Tadpole Club—as in being a bit of a Pied Piper with all the children following. Chris made the whole environment so much fun, with lots of different things to do. Besides using all the playground equipment, the boys would be making things in the sandpit, or inside playing with Lego for hours. I would give out ice-creams and the whole environment would be relaxed and enjoyable.

An inquisitive mind was also a big part of Chris's personality. For example, he would buy can openers and radiograms from the school fete and then would pull them apart at home. He wanted to see how they were wired together and how they worked. Chris was always clever with his hands.

Chris had a very sensitive side and when he was watching *Dot and the Kangaroo* he would become emotional, crying his eyes out and would have to leave the room when Dot had to release the kangaroo back into the wild.

I wanted the boys to experience the love of dogs, just as I had during my childhood. My beloved chihuahua Minnie had eventually passed away at the ripe old age of fourteen while I was pregnant with Matthew, so I had been a few years without a dog. I knew it was essential that the boys were old enough to understand how to care for and keep a dog safe. Matthew was five and Chris seven when we got Micky, who was half King Charles Spaniel and half chihuahua.

Micky was the most beautiful dog and he became a treasured member of our family. He had so much go in him!

Chris was also a very enterprising little boy with a real entrepreneurial spirit. He used to set up shop in the shed and sell cakes and other things that he had made from his sandpit. Matthew would be his assistant and I would be their customer. Chris also ran raffles around our neighbourhood. Our neighbours all knew the type of nature Chris had and they were very supportive—when he knocked on their door, they would take the raffle very seriously. He handmade everything—all the tickets had numbers on them, and he had a little basket of different things which were the prizes. He earned real money from these raffles and one of our neighbours, Jan, made the comment, "Gee Chris is enterprising."

Always Chris was busy! He would come home from school and you wouldn't hear much from him as he would go straight out to play. Chris never stopped inventing and building. He loved the excitement of Christmas, but the aftermath wasn't easy for him. Chris would get extremely depressed after all the festivities had finished and I would find him sitting in the corner crying. I would have to direct his attention to looking forward to the next celebration, which was Easter. One Easter, when he was about six and Matthew was four, I looked outside, and Chris had constructed two crosses in our backyard—one for him and one for Matthew. Using light string, he had tied himself and Matthew onto the crosses. Chris wanted to recreate the death and resurrection of Jesus at Easter.

As a big brother, Chris was usually kind and helpful to Matthew. One time, I remember being out for a few hours and my mother was minding the boys. One of Matthew's first teeth was loose, and Chris may have been trying to help his brother to get it out. He took it upon himself to attach a string around the offending tooth and pulled it out! I came back to Matthew crying about his lost tooth! Matthew was his little mate, always right there beside Chris. They were very close, despite being so different in their personalities.

From when Matthew was two or three, it was clear that he was extremely bright, with a very analytical mind. Even if we were just having a conversation, he would be looking up at the ceiling and processing everything you were saying as it was being said. Matthew was also very observant. After a day at school, he would be able to tell me exactly what he and Chris needed for the next day. He was always correct, and it was very helpful for me. I would check the newsletter and sure enough Matthew was correct. I could always count on his bright and accurate memory for knowing what the boys needed at school. Matthew's ability to retain and remember lots of information was like the news bulletin!

Matthew was not as emotionally resilient as Chris, who had the ability to push through challenging situations. He was a very sensitive little boy and more introverted than Chris. He needed his own space and a lot more sleep than his older brother. Matthew also needed a lot more support and he didn't cope well with change. When he was four years old, Matthew started pre-school, attending two mornings and two afternoons a week. I needed to be aware of where he was at emotionally, so that he could settle properly. When it came time to leave, if I didn't keep full focus and eye contact with him as I was going, he would break down crying.

My sister used to say that Matthew was lucky I was his mother because I was able to understand his emotional needs very well. Matthew needed his environment to be safe and private and a good example of this was when he was learning to swim. His swimming lessons were in a complex and I used to have to arrange it so that the complex was free of any people other than his swimming instructor, himself and me. This helped Matthew relax enough so he could learn to swim. Once he learned how, he was a very good swimmer, and he also loved other sports such as tennis, golf and soccer.

One of Matthew's unique qualities was how straight to the point he could be with what he said. He was one of those children who spoke very well. For example, Chris would call my sister "Aunty Ree" and Matthew would correct him saying, "It's not Aunty Ree, it's Aunty Maree." I remember being at a service station getting petrol and I had the car windows down. A larger built lady walked past, and Matthew asked, "Why is that lady so fat?" Another time, we were waiting in line at the ladies' toilets in McDonald's for a long time and Matthew asked, "Is that lady in there doing a poo?" He was straight to the point, but his comments were never unkind. He was just telling things as he saw them in his four-year-old mind. As a mother, I could see clearly how observant he was at such a young age.

Both boys went to the local pre-school in Kaleen and when it came time for Christopher to begin school, Richard wanted him to attend the O'Connor Christian School. It was very important to Richard that the boys attended a Christian school and learn about God and the Bible. I did some research and O'Connor Christian School's policy was to take a percentage of Richard's salary to pay the fees. It was simply too much for us to afford and so I started looking around for other options. I looked down at Matthew, who was only two years old at the time, and thought I would have to go back to work if I agreed for Christopher to attend this Christian school. So, I asked Richard to allow Chris to go to St Joseph's Catholic School instead. This was quite a distance from our home in Kaleen and involved a lot of driving backwards and forwards to this school because they had to go out of area. The local Catholic school had no vacancies for children who weren't Catholic.

Chris started Kindergarten and he seemed quite nervous and was blinking his eyes a lot. I volunteered for canteen duty, helped with reading for his class and on stalls at the fete. Chris was the fourth youngest in his class and he was struggling. I kept a close watch on him to make sure he was coping but I couldn't move him to another class because it was a one-stream school. Chris has a nature to push through, never complaining and wanting to please.

When I was on canteen duty, he would come over with his so-called friends and I would give them all ice-creams. They were only using Chris though, because when I looked out the window, I could see them snatch the ice-creams off him and run away. Even though Chris never came back and told me, I knew he was getting bullied! And although I was unable to confirm this, my belief was that the bullying was the root cause of a lot of the problems he was experiencing at school.

Chris's teacher believed his difficulties at school were due to his being a slow learner. We tried many different things to assist him, including eye glasses, balancing on a board for coordination, spending hours at home helping him with his reading and doing everything else we could think of. It seemed endless and nothing was working. Chris battled on from Kindergarten until the end of Grade 2.

I was at Chris's parent/teacher interview when I told his teacher I was thinking of having him repeat Grade 2. This was going to put Chris as the third eldest in the class and I was hoping that this would break the cycle of abuse and bullying. The teacher wasn't convinced this was the way to go but I decided it was worth a try! She would often say that Chris would grow up to be the "salt of the earth". At the time, I didn't really understand what she meant by this, but it seemed that she was saying a good thing. Those who are the "salt of the earth" are worthy of respect, because they can deal with difficult or demanding situations without making any unnecessary fuss. This was certainly true of Christopher.

And so, at the beginning of the next school year, Chris started Grade 2 all over again. He stood at the end of the line next to his old classmates who were moving up to Grade 3. Chris was brave and compliant, and he pushed through without a word. I knew he would be feeling it deep within. I found the day to be emotional and very difficult because, besides what was happening with Christopher, it was also Matthew's first day at St Joseph's, in the Kindergarten class. He was not coping at all—screaming, crying and refusing to leave me. The teachers were trying to console him, even taking him to see his big brother in class. I introduced him to a group of other little boys and told him their names, but nothing made any difference to his level of distress. There was no way he was going to stay if I left! To help him settle, I decided to stay with Matthew for the first thirty minutes of his day and take his little group for reading. I did this for the first twelve months of his schooling, and this made all the difference to Matthew being able to make some good solid friendships, which in turn made all the difference to his experience at school.

Matthew grew to love his time at St Joseph's, becoming one of the most popular students in his class with his friends and teachers alike. At whole school assembly Matthew would often receive awards.

Chris was coping well with repeating Grade 2 and all the slow learning issues disappeared. Because I was very active in the school, I could see that he was making genuine friends. I was relieved that the decision I had made for Chris to repeat was the right one for his emotional wellbeing. Instead of just surviving, he was now thriving.

With Matthew and Christopher both enjoying their years at St Joseph's and doing very well emotionally and academically, I was starting to feel more relaxed.

I was concerned that the boys might feel rejected due to the segregation between Catholic and non-Catholic children at St Joseph's. Not being Catholic meant that Chris and Matthew were only allowed to watch and not participate in their first Holy Communion and Confirmation. I thought that over time—all their primary school years—this might cause psychological damage. I rang the local priest at St Joseph's and explained my concerns to him, but he was from the old school and I don't think he appreciated being challenged! He rudely responded that these children were too young to decide to become a Catholic and then he hung up on me! Like a dog with a bone, I was very determined, and I refused to give up on this issue. I decided to ring the parish priest at St Michael's school in

Kaleen where only Catholic children were accepted. He was a younger priest and I thought he might be more receptive.

I made an appointment and he came around to our home one evening when the boys were asleep. I don't believe either of us knew what we were getting ourselves into as we discussed and debated the issue for hours. I refused to accept that Chris and Matthew could not be included in St Joseph's spiritual programs. This young, understanding priest and I could not come to an agreement. I kept saying that if Jesus was here today, He would not look at my boys and reject them. I would not back down on this issue and allow Chris or Matthew to be damaged psychologically over what I saw as stupid religious doctrines. The priest tried to explain things to me, but I honestly couldn't understand what he was saying. After all, I had no understanding of the Catholic faith—or, for that matter, any faith. Nor did I see any reason why I would need to have a faith.

I had no real belief in God, and I think for me the issue was more a human justice rather than a religious one. I have always had a strong sense of justice and during my own school days I would always befriend the child who was lonely or picked on. I think I was a fighter for fairness for others and this seemed to be a similar case for me—only much more important because it involved my own children!

Richard was absent during this time of discussion and debate. He did not seem to care about helping me to sort out an issue I was so clearly passionate about. Maybe he thought I was fighting a losing battle—that there was no way I could possibly win against the Catholic Church. He had also quietened down a lot from his earlier born-again experience and he was home more often. He still read his Bible but—much to my relief—he was no longer trying to convert me!

It was getting close to midnight when this kind young Catholic priest threw his hands in the air and told me to bring Chris and Matthew around to him every second Thursday. I think he was worn down by my determined nature and refusal to give in! The boys were able to attend an after-school program called an RCIA (Rite of Christian Initiation for Adults), which was adapted for children. Neither of the boys seemed to mind attending this simple and easy program on how to become a Catholic. In due course, I was able to inform St Joseph's that, in the eyes of the church, the boys were recognised as Catholic. They could now participate fully in the school's spiritual program!

Christopher was past the age of first Holy Communion so, with the lovely young priest officiating, he was confirmed in a big Catholic service at St Michael's church which Richard and I attended as a family. I don't think Richard ever realised what a fight I had put up so that our Anglican sons could finally be included in the Catholic spiritual program at St Joseph's. Matthew was still young enough to do his first Holy Communion back with his school friends at St Joseph's.

The fight was worth it as the spiritual program proved to be a wonderful experience for the boys. For the remainder of their primary school years, Chris and Matthew were able to take Holy Communion and regularly attend church. Matthew was often asked to do a reading, because he was an above average reader, and this was a very special privilege.

Our family holidays were something else we enjoyed. We often took Chris and Matthew away during the school holidays and sometimes extended the time to three to four weeks, with really good friends who had three children. This was an exciting time for us all as we enjoyed swimming in the pool where we were staying or going to the beach. I was always delighted to hear the five children playing together outside and at night-time they loved playing board games together. Our husbands would always cook us fabulous barbecues and my girlfriend and I enjoyed our quality time with each other. These were magical holidays for us all because we loved each other's company. Richard would build sandcastles and was a fabulous loving father. Our favourite coastal holiday destinations were Coffs Harbour, The Entrance and the Gold Coast. These were great holidays, and both Chris and Matthew have fantastic memories of them.

I also really wanted to give Chris and Matthew the opportunity to experience camping, so after having some time in a holiday house with them, my sister and I would stay together after Richard returned for work and we set up camp. Richard didn't want to do any camping and I respected that. Richard was always concerned when he was leaving. He would always say to me, "Don't turn your back on the ocean." He knew how quickly the ocean could turn, and he was worried about Chris and Matthew. I enjoyed my childhood camping and I wanted to seize the moment and give the boys a different experience. These experiences were usually down the south coast in the Mollymook, Ulladulla and Narooma region. All these holidays were the most bonding years of my married and family life, never to be forgotten.

Chapter 6
Someone to Believe Me

To the outside world, it appeared as though our family life was picture-perfect. However, Richard and I were constantly under financial pressure and I never had my own spending money. I was so anxious that I would write down everything I spent money on, even down to a cup of coffee. If I wanted something like a mascara, I would have to get it as part of my big grocery shop and hide it from him. We had a bankcard, but Richard would not allow my name to be on it. I didn't have access to use it, and nor was I able to withdraw any money from bank accounts. I found it hard to comprehend Richard's need to have control of all our finances. I was also a good saver and managed my own money well prior to getting married.

My mother was very generous. I didn't realise it at the time, but the boys and I were always dressed in whatever she bought for us. I was so grateful for her help that I didn't think to question this. Looking back, my mother was propping us up. Because she bought beautiful things for us and I was too young to understand what was happening, I didn't realise I had a major problem with Richard's behaviour towards money. He never allowed us to have a joint bank account and he would only give me $20 a month spending money. I was expected to save up for things I wanted or needed.

I wanted to buy a flyscreen door. I knew that the only way I could do this was to go back to work. I was a self-motivated person and very organised and I took on five different part-time jobs. I did marketing jobs for Newham Security Systems and for the National Gallery, where I interviewed people for certain exhibitions. I provided respite care for people with Alzheimer's Disease where I would get them into and out of bed and take them on picnics, chasing after them when they ran away. I was quite offended when I was told to stop giving 120% to these people when 90% would do. I gave over and above what was required of me. I oversaw catalogue distribution for Progress Press—with stores like Target and Grace Brothers—on the north side of town. I would go around all the distributors and check that they were doing their areas correctly, as well as covering any necessary shifts. My fifth and final part-time job was demonstrating a cell skincare range of non-animal-tested cleansers and moisturisers in David Jones. All these jobs revolved around Richard's work hours or on the weekend when he would be home to mind Chris and Matthew.

I was very busy with my part-time jobs, running the house and taking the boys to tennis, soccer and swimming lessons.

I knew something was wrong when I began experiencing head spins and feelings of dizziness. I made an appointment to see my GP and explained my symptoms to him. He wrote me out a script for an anti-depressant and even though I told him I didn't feel depressed, he asked me to trust him and take the medication. I never got the prescription filled; instead I ripped it up. Looking back, I realised the GP had not asked me what I was doing in my life and so he didn't know how busy I was. He also failed to explain what was causing my head spins.

I decided that, instead of all my part-time jobs, I needed just one regular job. I wanted to go back to work because I had resigned myself to the fact that I would not be having any more children. It wasn't that I was wanting a third child in the hope that the baby might be a girl, but that I had always wanted to have three children. Even though I desperately wanted a third baby, Richard was adamant that we were only having the two. So, I gave away all of Matthew's baby clothes and began to work through my grief.

I applied for one of two administrative positions within the government. I told Richard that applying for the job would be good practice for the future. I didn't expect to get an interview because I had been out of the Public Service for years. I had filled out the application form but failed to address the selection criteria. When I enquired about my application, I was informed of this and was given twenty-four hours to rectify it, and Richard and I worked on my revised application together.

With over 100 people applying for the position, I was amazed and excited when my husband took the phone call to inform me I had been successful in my application. I had secured the first administrative position and the hours were 8.00 am until 1.30 pm, Monday to Friday. This was perfect for me. Richard could put the boys on the bus, and I would be there to get them off the bus at 3.00 pm. I would also be able to resign from my five part-time jobs, which was a big relief.

On Orientation Day, I arrived on time, ready to find out all the information about what the job would entail. The second successful applicant—who was to take on afternoon shift—was already there. She was an older woman and her daughter and sister already worked in the Department. I sensed that a conversation had already taken place and that something was not quite right. Sure enough, there had been some changes made, of which I was unaware. The position was no longer in Security and had been switched to Building Management. The other lady was not happy with all the afternoon shifts and she wanted me to work her afternoon shift five days a fortnight from 1.30 pm until 6.00 pm. I was so intimidated by her and the Building Management team and I ended up caving into their demands and working half morning and half evening shifts.

I was very upset, and I rang my husband to explain what had happened. I was distraught, wondering what I could do about the boys. Richard was not supportive at all.

"After school and in school holidays it's your problem!" was his angry response to this dilemma.

Once again, my husband had left it to me to solve a problem that affected our whole family. Looking back, all I wanted and needed was his support and reassurance that we could discuss this later at home that night. I was only thirty-three years old and naïve, not realising that I had the option to decline the position. The terms offered were not those which I had applied—and been accepted—for.

So, I accepted the job, believing it was the only way to ease some of the financial pressure we were under. At 3.00 pm every day when I was at work, I would feel sick in the stomach because I was not there to meet Christopher and Matthew at the bus. I had asked my sister and my mum to help and be with the boys from 3.00 pm but they both were unavailable. My dear friend Leanne, whom I had known since we were two years old, came to my rescue. I didn't want to impose on her as she had two very active children of her own, Jodie and Gary, but I had no other option available to me.

I began to develop severe pain. I had started the job in June 1990 and after eight months, the pain was constant and mirrored the symptoms of gallstones or pancreatitis. I had no idea what was causing this or what was happening to me. I didn't tell anyone about my health problems and, thinking I had indigestion or a virus, I kept running to the chemist for something to help. I was confused because the pain I experienced was like the gallbladder attacks. Since I had already had my gallbladder removed, I knew that this couldn't possibly be the reason for the pain.

I went on holidays in early March 1991 with our friends and their children. I couldn't eat or drink much without experiencing pain, but I found after about four days away from the work place I was able to start drinking and eating again without it causing distress and pain. I returned home from three weeks of holiday and went back to work, and all my abdominal pains and cramps came back. I wasn't aware that working the afternoon shift in my job and being unavailable to get my little boys off the bus was causing this pain. I also didn't understand how the emotional can affect the physical. I was at a loss as to why I was in constant pain with such severe spasms in the stomach.

Christopher and Matthew were now eleven and eight years old. The pain I had been experiencing became so excruciating that I had no choice but to go to the hospital. The doctors thought I might have Crohn's Disease and I was referred to a gastroenterologist, who asked me what I thought was wrong with me. I knew it wasn't my gallbladder, as this had been removed when I was twenty. An ERCP—An Endoscopic Retrograde Cholangiopancreatography—was organised. This is a medical technique that employs a combination of fluoroscopy and endoscopy to diagnose and treat disorders affecting the biliary tree or pancreatic ducts. It is a medically risky procedure, but the specialist believed it was the best course of action because he wanted to see if there were any stones in my bile ducts. I also had a colonoscopy, endoscopy, pancreatitis check, a bowel check to see if there was anything wrong with my stools and a procedure to see if my blood was clotting properly.

I was extremely anxious about all these procedures and I started dry retching due to the stress of not knowing what was wrong with me, as well as the excruciating pain I was in. The specialist was quite young and said the procedures were urgent but then had failed to follow through, putting someone else in before me. I waited too long in a state of extreme anxiety. Finally, I was admitted to hospital and all the invasive tests were performed. Everything came back normal and, without consulting me, the specialist came to the wrong conclusion that my problems were psychosomatic. In one day, I was given three doses of a very powerful drug, liquid Haloperidol. This is a typical antipsychotic medication, used in the treatment of schizophrenia, nausea and vomiting, delirium, agitation and acute psychosis. It seemed harmless enough when I was given it and was like having a little drink of water. Because I was only thirty-three and in a medical ward in hospital, I trusted the doctors and the treatment they were prescribing for me. I hadn't been told what medication they were giving me.

I was talking to my friend Leanne when the next thing I knew, my whole jaw had locked, my head spasmed and jerked and my whole body was twisted. I went from standing upright to being in a completely contorted position. The three doses of the Haloperidol must have built up in my bloodstream. I was given two choices by the doctors—I could either go home or be admitted to the Psychiatric Ward. I knew I couldn't go home. I was not coping with the intense pain and I thought if I went to the Psychiatric Ward, I could sort out what had gone wrong.

After being admitted, I was given Cogentin to reverse the effects of the Haloperidol. My right eye, the side of my face and head were all still affected—and to this day I still get spasms from being given the Haloperidol. Some people have died as a result of being given this very powerful drug. Even though my face was spasming and I was in such pain, my mind was still intact. I decided that I would not fall into line by taking any other medication they wanted to give me. I would pretend to swallow the medication but would instead spit it out. By this stage, I had lost all trust in the doctors and their drugs and weird side effects.

I said in my spirit, "Lord, someone please believe me". The neuralgia that was going through my face, throat and teeth was absolutely agonising, but it was a long time before I was able to be diagnosed. For months, I would travel to any chronic pain group I could find.

At first, Richard was sympathetic to my illness but then after a while, he became very hard and indifferent towards me. Christopher and Matthew were still so young, being only eleven and eight, and

Richard was totally frustrated by my continued ill-health. Our marriage had been so happy for the first fifteen years and, as far as I was concerned, everything seemed good.

Now I had gone from being capable and running everything smoothly to being totally unwell and barely able to function. I was trying to be a good mother, but this was hard because I was in agony. My mother-in-law Dorothy came across to help. I would go to my sister Maree's place, lie in a spare bed and just rock from the agony I was in. I used to ring for the ambulance a lot as my throat muscles would go weak internally. It felt as though my throat was collapsing but, as I found out later, it was because the nerves were damaged, and I was having extreme muscle spasms.

Through one of the chronic pain groups I attended, I met a wonderful lady who was able to secure an appointment for me to see the ex-Superintendent of Calvary Hospital. The blood was pooling in my legs and he sent me to see a Vascular Physician at St Vincent's Private Hospital in Sydney. Finally, I had a referral away from my home town, where I was not believed—even by my mother, my sister, my husband, extended family and most of my close friends. Not being believed by those close to me was devastating for me. The earlier whisper of, "Lord, someone please believe me," became like a mantra. I said it over and over in my mind and heart because I was desperate and couldn't find anyone who would believe me. From December 1991 until October 1992 I would say this repeatedly. Finally, the good Lord did send someone to believe me!

A doctor at St Vincent's took blood tests and agreed that I could be right; that I was, in fact, very ill and not just imagining things. He sent me to see Dr Garrick, a top neurologist who told me no psychiatric patient could possibly make up what I told him was happening to me. He had me admitted to St Vincent's under the care of himself and Dr McGrath, a Vascular Physician. I went through this hospitalisation on my own, even though my sister and her second husband, Laurie, brought my father to see me. This turned out to be a useless and heartbreaking visit as they stayed not ten minutes before my father was taken to the nearest drinking hole. The grog had got him, which was typical of his behaviour by this stage of his life.

Dr McGrath and Dr Garrick worked with me for ten days and I was given some sort of diagnosis of glossopharyngeal neuralgia/neuropathic pain. There was a right hemi cranial headache with pain extending into the right side. Even though there was no cure for my condition, I was much more settled emotionally and felt validated and respected because someone finally believed me.

I stayed under the care of Dr Garrick for the next few decades and was also diagnosed with hemifacial dystonia. Dr Garrick said on numerous occasions that Haloperidol did me no good. I knew exactly what he meant. Due to the threat of possible litigation, we were unable to say much more.

Even though I felt validated and respected, I had hit rock-bottom. When I rang Richard, he wasn't nice to me and I felt alone. Even though I felt such wonderful relief to finally be believed, within myself I had never been lower. I felt no emotion whatsoever. I could have walked out of that hospital and been run over and not cared. I had become a shell of my former self.

Chapter 7

Born Again

I was lying in my hospital bed when I heard a soft, still voice saying, "Go and find a quiet spot." I got up and the first place I went was a loungeroom. It wasn't quiet, as many cleaners were talking there. I continued searching for a quiet spot and caught the lift down to the little chapel on the next floor. No one came in and no one went out. I had found my quiet spot!

I sat in silence in that little chapel. I didn't pray at that time because I didn't believe there was a God. An hour-and-a-half had passed, and as I got up and opened the door to leave the chapel, I heard that same soft, still voice say, "Thank the Lord for belief." This was what I had been crying out for since December 1991 and it was now October 1992, almost a full year later! This was my revelation of a God!

I felt no excitement and I told nobody because I was still so numb inside from all that had happened to me. I knew I had to go home to my children and running the household, but I was feeling low from being in severe nerve pain and from knowing there was no cure for my condition. I was tired of having an indifferent husband and I did not want the Christian God that he believed in to be the same God who had spoken to me. I decided to keep the experience of God speaking to me all to myself as I could not have coped with any more disbelief from others. I knew the God who spoke to me believed me, as did Dr Garrick. This was my only consolation at this very painful and challenging time.

I was physically unwell, but I still wanted to nurture my family by preparing wholesome homecooked meals for them. This required a massive effort, as I was in so much pain from the neuralgia which affected my neck, jaw, teeth and the area near my tonsils. I would begin the meal preparation at 9.00 am, and by the time Richard and the boys arrived home, the evening meal would be ready. The plates would be lined up, filled with good fresh food which needed only reheating.

Richard was not happy about this. To him, the reheating created a drama because the food hadn't been dished up straight from the pot!

I remember one day I was, as usual, struggling just to peel pumpkin and I thought listening to some music might help. Maree had given me some Maranatha Christian music tapes, but—even though God had spoken to me—I consciously chose not to listen to them. I told myself, "No Christian music." I turned the radio on to 2CC, a mainstream station that played 70s music. The music that was coming through the radio had a typical 70s beat, but the lyrics were unusual and caught my attention. They were saying, "You've got to serve somebody." I didn't really know what that meant but I believe God was trying to speak to me through those lyrics. I don't know how this song came to be on the radio. I never touched the dials of the radio, but I heard them announce this was Radio Rhema, the Christian station. Radio Rhema was on very intermittently, about once every three weeks, and it was also hard to tune into it properly.

God was trying to catch my attention, but I was still not wanting to have anything to do with the Christian God that Richard believed in.

Because I was in so much pain, my mother was convinced that I needed something like hypnotherapy or to learn meditation. I was in the local bakery and I saw a pamphlet advertising a talk by Sri Chinmoy, who was described as a spiritual master and teacher of meditation. His talk was in the city, but I got there late and found that the doors were closed, and no one could get in. I believe now that this was God's way of wanting to divert me away from false spiritual teachings.

However, the next day Sri Chinmoy was at the Belconnen Community Centre. I decided to attend the lunchtime meeting and when I walked in, I noticed a large photo of an Eastern religious man—Sri Chinmoy—on display and lots of people already sitting down. I had a knowing within myself that this wasn't the right God, but I still stayed.

When I finished the meditation, I walked out of the room and I noticed a servery with a sign saying, *Eat what you like, pay what you want.* A young man of around thirty was behind the counter and he asked me where I had been. I replied that I had been at Sri Chinmoy, but I didn't really know much more than that. It was of no concern to me when he said I shouldn't have gone there as it wasn't the right God. He asked me if I would like some prayer, but my reply was, "No thank you, I'm all prayed out."

I left the building intending to go home, but just as I got to the car park, I suddenly changed my mind. I went back to the young man and said, "If that prayer is still for the offering, I think I will have some."

The young man was joined by a more mature lady, who would have been in her fifties, and they both prayed over me. As they prayed, I experienced a strong heat and a light, unlike anything I had ever known before. I had a revelation that I was receiving the Christian God, the one true God of the Bible. Even though I was totally opposed to the God Richard believed in, and had been so damaged by his conversion, I knew that what I was receiving was the truth. It was a real revelation of God!

"Where am I?" I asked, and they told me that I was at an outreach run by Ecumenical Christians.

I returned home, but I kept what had happened to myself. I was so confused about who God was. Because I'd had such a positive experience with the young Catholic priest at St Michael's, I thought he could help. He had made such an impression on me with his kindness and I felt drawn to him. If it weren't for the fact that we had that earlier discussion over my children missing out on the sacraments, I might not have felt comfortable reaching out to him.

I decided I would start attending St Michael's church and I went three mornings a week, listening to the young priest's short sermons. I couldn't receive Communion because I wasn't a Catholic. During this time, I met a lady called Ines who also lived in Kaleen. She was a more mature lady and she took me under her wing, becoming like a mother figure for me. Ines was kind, gentle, soft and encouraging and I felt safe with her. This was important for me, as I had lost all my confidence.

For the next twelve months, I went everywhere with her and I continued to attend St Michael's parish services. I then found that the young Catholic priest was born again and was running a charismatic service on a Saturday night, which Ines also encouraged me to attend.

I stayed under the guidance and teaching of this young priest for quite a while and eventually I decided I wanted to receive Communion, so I went to the RCIA (Rite of Christian Initiation of Adults). Richard didn't seem to mind all of this. He had lost some of his early passion for the Lord and was now at a different stage of faith to me. He appeared quite blasé about me attending church. He was also struggling to cope with work and with the fact that, as a wife, I could no longer physically perform all the duties that I had once been able to do.

Richard was also very angry that the government department I had been with when I became ill had not taken any responsibility for the bullying I was subjected to. Therefore, he left the well-paid position he had been in, took a package and decided to stay home. I was under the impression Richard did this so we could have our house paid off and spend quality time together. This was not to be. Instead, he started to build a compensation case over my being bullied in the workplace. Workplace bullying was unheard of in those days, but Richard wanted someone to take responsibility for what I went through, so he took on the department I was working for. My original job agreement had specified my hours would be 8.00 am to 1.30 pm, but then I had been forced to job share the position and do afternoons as well. Even though I was a great advocate where others (especially my children) were concerned, I was hopeless about entering any conflict on my own behalf.

For six years, the boys and I watched Richard work on my compensation case, battling for justice. It was horrendous for us as a family, and I was very concerned for Richard's mental health as he was determined to fight this battle to the bitter end. He would work on the computer around the clock—up all night and most of the day, as well as helping me with the general running of our home. Even though he was still very much a hands-on father, Richard struggled to relate to me.

I thought back to the time when Richard had decided we would be having only two children. Some women I knew at the time were getting pregnant without consulting their husbands but I did not want to be deceptive and so I respected Richard's decision. There are choices we make for others that are not in our own best interests and this was how I now felt about not having a third baby. I couldn't help wondering how different my life would now be had I gone ahead and had a third child. Having a third child meant I would not have applied for the job; I would not have been bullied and I would also still be in a happy marriage to Richard. I felt we were happy until the workplace bullying took place. I thought I would also still be in good health because I knew, beyond a shadow of a doubt, that the high doses of Haloperidol that I was given—and the horrendous reaction to it—had caused the devastation to my autonomic nervous system.

While Richard was busy trying to get me compensation for being bullied in the workplace, I was busy trying to understand the Christian faith. I got very involved in St Michael's Catholic Church and did the Lenten program leading up to Easter. This is a program for groups or individuals that provides a process for reflection and discussion on the Sunday scriptures during Lent. I was part of a group of ladies doing the program. It went on to become a Bible study/sharing group, where I was able to develop some close friendships. I also found out that the young priest believed in full immersion baptism. Richard told me I was being ridiculous to think that a Catholic priest would do this. He got the shock of his life when the young priest arranged to borrow someone's swimming pool, and at 8.30 in the morning, I was re-baptised by full immersion. I became a Catholic in the eyes of the Catholic Church. Richard had been where I now was back in 1981—ten years earlier—but he was now in a very different stage of faith. He was not happy for me that we now shared a Christian faith but instead was indifferent to the fact that I had been born again and that I still wasn't well. I was now the one doing what Richard had done years before—going to the Christian bookshop, buying the Christian books and putting up the plaques in the boys' room. It was driving both him and the boys crazy. They had been very young when Richard had accepted Jesus into his heart but now that they were much older it was very confronting for them to see this happen to me.

I was reading scripture and listening to *Keys to Successful Living* by Derek Prince on the radio. When the weather was nice, I would drive to the lake and sit by myself, reading my Bible. If the weather was harsher, I would go to the chapel at Calvary Hospital to do the same. Being in these secluded places was the only way I could get away from Richard and have privacy to read my Bible without feeling guilty.

I could not get enough of reading the Bible and it became alive to me! The Holy Spirit was revealing things and I was understanding without someone teaching me. I understood the Shepherd was Jesus and the sheep were the people, and that He was the bridegroom and the bride was the church—the people of God. This understanding came to me supernaturally and the more I read the Bible, the more my faith grew. I was feeling uplifted by the services I was attending and being under the guidance and teaching of this young Catholic Charismatic priest was instrumental in helping me grow in Jesus. I was finding peace in my spirit which I could not get at home while Richard was fighting the compensation case. Even though my body wasn't getting any better, my mind and my human spirit were getting stronger. Through Ines, I was also becoming stronger emotionally.

Richard, however, was becoming weaker through fighting the compensation case. It was tearing us apart as a family. I decided to make an appointment for both of us to see my neurologist, Dr Garrick, in Sydney. I hoped that the consultation would help Richard understand my condition and that, as a result, we could become closer. Christopher and Matthew came with us. The appointment was literally five minutes from where we were staying but Richard wouldn't allow us to take a taxi. We had to use public transport. This was very difficult for me physically, but Richard couldn't comprehend how it would have made things so much easier to just catch a taxi.

During the consultation, Richard told Dr Garrick about the compensation case. The doctor was very concerned and explained to Richard that he disagreed with fighting government authorities. Dr Garrick said that, regardless of whether you win, these cases can break you emotionally. He explained to us that the injuries I had received to the autonomic nervous system were equivalent to being hit by a bus. He said that what I was dealing with was so difficult that I could develop mental health issues, or turn to alcohol for comfort, or end up in an institution. He said I might even think of taking my own life.

Something rose in my spirit when Dr Garrick said this to Richard! I thought there is no way any of these things are going to happen to me because I have God in my life now. God knew my heart and He would give me the strength to push through!

I clung onto and memorised scripture verses that spoke to my heart and believed God was carrying me through. "I can do all things through Christ who strengthens me." (Philippians 4:13)

Dr Garrick also explained that there was no firm diagnosis for my condition, and that this made it very difficult for people to understand what I was going through.

I wished I had a more easily identifiable disease! I thought maybe then Richard would show me some compassion and understanding. Instead, he became even harder and tougher on me. My hope that the consultation would bring us closer together was dashed.

Unfortunately, it changed nothing.

Chapter 8

Disharmony

W e came home to Kaleen, and Richard and I continued in a
very difficult marriage. Richard was utterly driven by the
compensation case, blaming the government department for the loss
of my health. Considering my physical condition and the pain I was
in, his expectations on me as a wife and mother were very unrealistic.
Still, I wanted to make our marriage work! For example, I bought a
book on what it takes to make a successful marriage. Even though it
was an easy read, Richard was not the slightest bit interested in it. I
also tried to inject some romance into the marriage by booking a
cruise for us, so that the two of us could get away and spend some
quality time together. I ended up losing the deposit of $400 because
Richard told me he was not going to do anything with me until
"things were perfect". I knew this was an impossibility, especially
because there was no work being done to sort out any of our marital
problems.

I remember wanting Richard to come with me to see *Sense and
Sensibility* at the movies. Predictably, he refused. Even though I had
never been out on my own on a Saturday night before, I was
determined to go. Richard was adamant that he would not be
accompanying me. I was just putting the finishing touches to my
makeup when Richard came into the bathroom and told me he
would put himself out and come with me. My reply was that I was

not a charity case and off I went on my own. After all, I had asked him all day to come with me.

It being a Saturday night, the movie theatre was very crowded, mostly with couples. As I was standing in line waiting to purchase my ticket, I had to keep repeating to myself that it was okay to be on my own. I sat and enjoyed watching the movie and after it was over, I did a fist pump and said "Yes!" I was so proud of myself! I had finally conquered my fear of going out on my own.

During this time of marital strain and being so unwell with relentless nerve pain, one thing that kept me stable and sane was my women's group. These were the new friends I had made through the church. We would meet every Tuesday for Bible study/sharing, have lunch, celebrate one another's birthdays and support one another. They knew I was struggling and would make casseroles for extra food for us as a family. So many of my friends from my days as a young mother had by now fallen away, and I felt very blessed to have these beautiful compassionate new women in my life.

Richard's resentment towards me was growing. He resented me for my poor health, for the strain of the compensation case and even because I had come from a family where I was financially secure. His poor treatment of me was increasing and was about to escalate to a whole new—and very disturbing—level. One summer's night, Chris was mowing the lawns at my next-door neighbour Kath's place while Matthew and I were in the family room. As had become the norm, Richard spoke down to me about something.

I responded with, "Don't you dare speak to me like that!"

He came after me and put his hands around my throat, saying, "You poor little rich girl!"

I felt so shocked by this! I was already very weak from the hemifacial dystonia affecting the right side of my face and neck and then Richard hit me through the left arm and left side of my head. I was screaming but knew to not speak back at him as only silence would quieten his anger and frustration down.

After this happened, Richard told me he didn't expect me to sleep with him that night. He slept with Matthew in our bed and I took Matthew's bed. At 5.00 am I awoke from my sleep, feeling broken from the assault. Not just my body felt violated but also my mind, emotions and spirit. I said to the Lord, "I submit my spirit to you." I wanted to die.

And then I heard the soft, still voice again, telling me, "Don't let him rob you."

I knew God was speaking to me! This was enough to get me out of my son's bed and into the shower, so I would be ready to go and meet my friends at my Tuesday group.

I never mentioned anything to the group at the time, but afterwards I visited the young Catholic priest and spoke to him about what had happened. We prayed together about forgiveness and I knew Richard was in great distress over the breakdown of my health and the compensation case. The pressure he was under was extreme and caused him to snap. I wasn't making excuses for the behaviour but this was not in his character and he was deeply remorseful. I made a decision that our family needed to stay together and I desperately wanted to live and stay with my sons.

Christopher was about to finish Year 6 at St Joseph's. It was very clear to me that we could not afford a private school education for him, so Richard and I went to look at the local public high school together. Neither of us was impressed, but the location was convenient, with the school oval facing our house. On the day we looked at the new school, I noticed that my leg was sort of dragging and it felt weak. This wasn't obvious to anyone else and my neurologist, whom I was seeing every six months at this stage, put it down to a problem with my circulation. I was unwell, and Richard was fighting the compensation case. Given our circumstances, we felt we really had no other option but to make the difficult decision to put Chris into Kaleen High. Matthew could stay at St Joseph's for a further two years, until he finished Year 6, and we were very grateful to be able to manage this.

When Chris started at Kaleen High, it quickly became evident that he was extremely popular. Every morning, around 8.30 a.m., there would be at least fifteen or twenty boys, from in and around Kaleen, coming to our house so they could go to school with Chris. The big group he was part of was the most popular one in school and for the first six months, Richard and I were pleased with how Chris was going. Then we started to notice that he was changing. He would talk about how different it was being at a very big public school when he had been used to attending a very small one-stream Catholic primary school.

It was hard for Chris to process the different culture of behaviour that he now was part of. One example of this was the "spit balls"—papier-mâché balls that all the boys formed in their mouths and would then spit out. Another example was Chris wanting to change his schoolbag from the Billabong branded one we bought him and wear one that looked cooler. He also became very conscious of his appearance. We had already paid $4000 for braces for his upper and lower teeth and had also arranged for Chris to have a couple of moles removed from his face. He had also bought his own hair clippers and he wanted an undercut, which was the trend at that time. All his friends wanted one too. Because I was trying to understand where Chris was coming from emotionally, I decided to learn how this was done. Chris and his friends would all line up in the shed, where I would cut their hair. Richard would be screaming that I wasn't a qualified hairdresser, but I didn't let this deter me. I would do all the undercuts for Chris and his friends and then for Matthew and the neighbourhood friends, giving them "Number 1s" or whatever they wanted.

As part of his change in behaviour, Chris also took up smoking. Again, I wanted to stay close to him emotionally and for us to still be able to talk, and so I allowed Chris to smoke in the home environment rather than have him go elsewhere. We had a beautiful outdoor gauzed room and that was where Chris and his friends would go. Richard was very distressed by the smoking and he wanted to ban it from our home, believing Chris was being a bad influence on Matthew. Richard and I responded very differently to our son smoking. I wanted to stay close to Chris emotionally and, even though I didn't want to approve of the behaviour, I was frightened I would lose Chris if we banned him from smoking at home. And even though the smoking was a problem, Chris's attitude towards us was still very kind, without any cheek or back answering.

While these worrying changes to Chris's behaviour were taking place, Matthew was still applying himself very well at St Joseph's. He was happy and popular but also very observant, taking notice of everything his big brother did. Even though Richard thought Chris was a bad influence on Matthew, I wasn't at all worried because I knew they were such different personalities. Chris was a risk taker while Matthew was more observant and would think of the consequences of his actions.

At around this time, Chris had also bought a CB radio which he installed in his bedroom. His call sign was "Rebel". Matthew observed this behaviour but did not get involved. I can't say the same for me! Because I was an extrovert and I loved people, I got into the CB radio just as much as Chris, calling myself "Suzie Q". Richard was not impressed at all! On several occasions, he would walk past Chris's bedroom and scream at me to "Grow up!" I would not allow his reaction to deter me. I saw the CB radio as a diversion from how unhappy and unwell I felt.

I was still really struggling with balancing and walking issues and had no idea why this was happening. Our home at Snowy Place was bedlam, with a steady stream of youth coming before and after school. I always encouraged the boys to be able to bring their friends home. It was so hectic, and I found it very hard, but I made myself cope as I always wanted the boys and their friends to feel at home. In this way, we were able to get Chris through Year 7. And as he was going into Year 8, a very special person was about to enter his life.

Matthew was outside playing ball when he came inside to let Chris know that there was a girl outside who wanted to see him. Linda was new to Kaleen High, and when she told Chris she couldn't find her way to the bus stop, he did the gentlemanly thing and politely walked with her. Chris did not see it, but I knew that Linda was just pretending she was lost because she wanted to check Chris out. When he returned home, I told him I thought Linda might like him. Chris's reply was, don't be so ridiculous; that you'd have to be Arnold Schwarzenegger as she was the hottest girl in school.

Linda was fourteen and Chris was fifteen when they got together. Over time, she started to come to our home and spend a lot of time with the four of us, often staying overnight. We enjoyed having Linda as part of our family as she was such a loving and easy-going girl. I felt she was the daughter I never had. Linda was very kind to Chris and would often be in his bedroom, folding his t-shirts and putting them away in his drawers. She worked at Kentucky Fried Chicken a few suburbs away and I used to drive her there and would often drop her back home to her parents.

By now, Matthew had finished Year 6 and he transferred across to Kaleen High. I was grateful that both boys had their formative years at St Joseph's, which held them in good stead to cope at Kaleen High. Matthew was popular at St Joseph's and he had left a very close-knit group of friends, so the move was emotionally quite difficult for him. I also struggled emotionally with Matthew's transfer to Kaleen High. I believed that if I hadn't got sick and had been able to keep working, Matthew could have gone on to Daramalan, a Catholic high school, with all his friends. Unlike Chris, he wasn't rebellious in any way, but he found it hard to get out of bed to go to school in the mornings. To encourage him, I would go into his room and open his curtains to let the sun shine in.

For the first twelve months, Matthew would miss two or three days out of the five. This did not worry me as he was very bright. I would say to him to go and play on the computer and then he could see some friends when they got home from school. When he did attend school, I either drove him there or he walked.

To add to the distress of that year was our beloved dog Micky's diagnosis of severe diabetes. At the age of eight, Micky had taken a turn for the worse and the vet told me I would have to let him go. I rang Kaleen High and asked for the boys to be let out of school early. They were waiting at the kerb for me and when I pulled up with my sunglasses on, Matthew knew I was coming with bad news about Micky. As a family, this event was very traumatic for us. It was one of the most emotional times for us all as a family because Micky was such a legend of a dog with so much energy in him. He was the best natured dog—the perfect family pet who always loved playing with Chris and Matthew. We went to the vet and, while Matthew and I waited, Chris went in with Micky while the vet put him to sleep. He wrapped Micky up and we were able to bring him home to bury him in the grave Richard had dug.

It was so very hard to lose Micky, and Matthew was struggling enough at the loss of my health and trying to deal with a new school. I felt he really needed another dog. Richard was away for the weekend and I was reading the local newspaper when I saw three puppies advertised for sale. They were twelve-week-old King Charles Cavaliers, located close by in Kaleen. I decided to take Matthew with me and check them out. One of the pups was named Nelson and Matthew took a special liking to him. I wanted Matthew to have him and, even though I believed Richard would be opposed to us getting another dog, I was determined to put Matthew's needs first.

I was very anxious trying to bring the subject up with Richard, whose reaction was as I expected. He was furious with me for taking Matthew to look at the puppies and was adamant that we would *not* be getting Nelson. It was around the time of Richard's birthday and

Matthew was so upset that he didn't wish his father a happy birthday. Even though Richard blamed me for Matthew's reaction, it was enough to make him change his mind and allow our son to have Nelson.

Nelson was a magnificent little dog and he came at a time when our family was in crisis. He was a real breath of fresh air and brought in so much love!

Chapter 9

A Place of My Own

I started doing voluntary work as a receptionist for some psychologists at Youth with a Mission (YWAM). My job was to man the phones and get the client files out. Part of the criteria for the job was that I had to commit to a 12-step recovery program once a week. Because I wanted the work, I agreed to this. I would attend the meetings and listen to people talk but it was so different for me that I thought I was on another planet! I definitely didn't think I needed this program for myself.

This little bit of voluntary work was good for me as it got me out of the house and gave me a break from home. Richard was still working day and night on the compensation case and it was affecting us all. At around this time, I could see Chris was lacking motivation. When I looked closely, I saw his pupils were dilated. Even though I had no experience with marijuana and didn't know what it smelled like, I suspected Chris was smoking it. We lived near some stormwater drains and I wondered whether that was where Chris and his friends would go to smoke bongs.

Richard was really distressed about Chris smoking and he wanted him away from the home. I could see that it was getting difficult for Chris to navigate life through the teenage years. To me, it was such a big responsibility to bring both of my boys safely through their teens and I wanted as much helpful information as possible. While I was working with the psychologists at YWAM, I took the opportunity to educate myself about marijuana—what it cost on the streets and what signs to look out for—for example, getting the munchies.

Chris was fourteen when he progressed to drinking alcohol. Early one morning, around 1.30 a.m., Richard and I got a call from the police to come and get Chris. He and two of his friends had been picked up for underage drinking. I got out of bed, feeling concerned for Chris, but Richard was so angry that he couldn't come. I went down to the station to collect Chris and one of his friends. The other boy's mother was collecting her son. Chris's behaviour was unusual for such a compliant child, but even though his behaviour was very worrying, his school grades were still good. One lovely surprise at this hard time was being rung up by Kaleen High to come to assembly as Chris was receiving an award for being the most gifted and talented student.

Linda and Chris's relationship was also a lovely part of our lives and they happily attended their school formal together. I was still having a lot of trouble balancing and walking properly. I wanted to see Chris and Linda and their friends where they were getting the photos done. I could only shuffle in the pair of high heeled shoes I wore for the occasion. My health was deteriorating more and more rapidly but I had no one to talk to or understand me. I had asked Richard to come with me to see everyone dressed up in their formal clothes, but he wasn't interested in doing anything with me. It was such a lonely existence but my unconditional love for both my children was what kept me going.

When I first got sick and had a seizure from the effects of Haloperidol I had been such an overprotective and worrying mother. Now I was a different person and things that used to worry me no longer did. When Chris was sixteen, he came home from school one day with some information about an opportunity for travelling in outback America. He had no expectations or demands that he would go but I thought this was such a wonderful opportunity for him to experience the trip of a lifetime. Prior to becoming so ill, the old me would have said no way could Chris go, but now I realised how fragile and short life is, and how sickness can come so easily. Richard was beside himself, asking how could we afford it? He could not comprehend how it was possible that the trip could ever be funded. My response was that where there's a will, there's a way, and I made the decision that I wanted Chris to have this experience of a lifetime.

I started to fundraise with chocolates, dollar for dollar, travelling to different shopping centres. I was a regular at the Dickson shops, outside Woolworths, at the Jamieson Centre outside Coles and outside Cooleman Court, Weston. Two of Chris's friends did the same and Chris often came with me and his friends to fundraise with the chocolates. We fundraised until we had the exact amount we needed. The chocolate company was astounded at how I took this on single-handedly. I was extremely motivated, and I ended up raising $6600 over eighteen months, of which the chocolate company took one half and Chris had the other half.

The fundraising was very humbling for me because I had always worked at good jobs before and now here I was, outside Woolworths and Coles, asking people for money to fund my son's excursion. My observation of people who were dressed up and drove nice cars was that they rarely gave, and the people who appeared to have nothing were usually generous. Later, I did some further fundraising for Paraquad and I had to be very careful with how I walked on the pavement. My feet could trip up so easily on the slightest unevenness in the pavement. Over time it was becoming harder and harder to be able to dress up and wear high heels. My mobility issues were creeping up on me and I had no idea why this was happening. It was quite insidious. I had my appointment at St Vincent's and came back home with still no answers.

Even though I was in pain and things were very strained with Richard, I tried to keep up the fun in life—using the CB radio, doing my YWAM voluntary work and getting Chris's trip to America funded.

The day came and off Chris went with his friends, trekking outback America. Those who didn't go would often pop around after school to see how the trip was going. All was going smoothly except once when Chris called home, needing an extra $100. Richard refused to give this but fortunately, my mum with her generous spirit came to the party and the money was transferred to Chris. I was getting so worn down with the reality that anything to do with money was such a battle with Richard.

Around this time, I saw a sale on golf clubs and thought Matthew, who loved sport—particularly golf—would really appreciate a set. I mentioned this to Richard, but he was opposed to the idea. He was adamant that Matthew would not be spending his money on golf clubs because he would be needing to buy a car in the future. Matthew would not even be old enough to drive for another four years, and I was very concerned that Richard was not understanding about Matthew's emotional needs. Matthew would be using his own money to pay for the golf clubs. I had made sure that both Chris and Matthew had their own bank accounts from when they were babies and I regularly banked money for them when they were gifted some for birthday or Christmas from family members.

I also wanted to lighten the heavy atmosphere in our family as I felt as though we were falling apart. I decided to contact Laurie, (my brother-in-law) and asked him if he could take Matthew to the golf shop sale. Even though I knew this would be distressing to Richard, I also knew that emotionally it would uplift Matthew. Matthew came home with a beginner's set of golf clubs in a beautiful red buggy and he wanted to bring the clubs into his bedroom. Due to Richard's reaction, I thought it better if Matthew didn't do this, so he left the golf clubs in the shed. It was very upsetting that he couldn't have his golf clubs in his room and enjoy the excitement of buying them.

Shortly before Chris was due to return home, Matthew came home with information about a school excursion to travel to Cooma. Even though he didn't want to go, I knew Matthew needed something exciting to look forward to. I noticed a special deal for a New Zealand trip where, if you were under a certain age, you could travel for a discount price as long as you were accompanied by adults. My sister and her husband were going to New Zealand within this time frame and I suggested Matthew could have his first plane flight and go with them. The cost of the excursion with the school to Cooma was the same price as sending Matthew to New Zealand.

Naturally there was another battle with Richard over spending money, but I really wanted Matthew to experience something special and I was grateful that he could go. My desire was strong to see my two sons experience travel and broaden their horizons. Besides this, things were not good in our home life and I wanted the boys to have a break from all the chaos!

Chris returned from America and he had thoroughly enjoyed his trip, and had much to tell us. He still says to this day it was one of the best experiences of his life. I felt overjoyed that I'd played a part in making this happen for him. My own life's disappointments had spurred me on to want my children to see life was still full of hope and adventure. I was now putting all my trust in God and I was realising life was a gift and it was to be embraced and lived well!

Richard was still working relentlessly around the clock to get compensation. For him, this was the only way he could cope with the downfall of my health but for me, it was so very distressing to watch my husband working so hard.

In 1997, Richard was delighted when we were finally granted compensation and he immediately took full control of this money. I was awarded $72,000, with $120,000 on death. It was determined that I had suffered 45% impairment, and this was what the compensation award was based on. For me, 45% was just the tip of the iceberg as I felt as though I had lost 70% function and that I was now living on

30% of the old me. How could I explain this to anyone when they were not living in my body? And while Richard was thrilled with the outcome, for me it had nothing to do with the money. I had lost so much of the enjoyment of life, and I was still experiencing spasms and constant nerve pain down my throat, as well as facial pain. There was no relief from it.

One morning, within six months of the compensation being awarded, I woke and mentioned the nerve pain I had in my face to Richard. In a quiet manner, he said, "I think it's time for you to go."

Silent tears began to run down my face but, at the same time, it was a bit of a relief because dealing with Richard's indifference towards me was so exhausting. Chris was now seventeen and Matthew was fifteen. Knowing I had to leave my family home, I began searching for a little townhouse that I could afford in my own suburb. There was nothing available in Kaleen and I had no choice but to go out to Gungahlin, which at that time was like going to the other end of the Earth. In 1998 there was nothing there but Woolworths, a club and a petrol station.

I was going through the newspaper about midnight and I found a lovely little townhouse in Amaroo, advertised as "a slice of Heaven for one lucky soul". I went to look at it and it was just beautiful. It was only four months old, virtually brand new, and no gardens had been established. I remember saying to myself, "If you don't like this, you won't like anything." It had everything I wanted, including three bedrooms—so there would be enough room for the boys. After I saw it, I went back and told Richard about it and he said, "Aren't you going to procrastinate?" I told him no—that if I didn't like this, I wasn't going to like anything.

In those days, securing a property was a simple procedure. Richard put down $1000 to take it off the market. The townhouse was mine. I had no furniture other than a double bed and an old floral sofa my sister lent me. This was without a doubt the lowest point in my life. I had lost my children, Nelson the dog and my family home that I built with Richard. Even though Richard wanted me to leave, at no stage did I believe the marriage was over. I believed that moving into my own place was the only way that our marriage could survive and that we would reconcile in the future. My sister and her husband were concerned that I hadn't sought any legal advice and so they took me to see a solicitor. I was experiencing severe anxiety over what the solicitor was saying I was entitled to and I was in fear of what Richard would say or do once he realised I had sought legal advice.

Richard made an appointment to see his own solicitor and he brought along a beautiful bottle of red wine for him. There was a stark contrast between how Richard and I were functioning at that time. He was in very good physical shape, whereas I was in a great deal of pain and struggling desperately with my mobility. I was so naïve that I did not realise that Richard had organised a property settlement and this was what the appointment was all about.

As I was about to sign the paperwork, the solicitor asked me, "Are you sure this is what you want?"

I didn't reply and proceeded to sign. Richard had made it very clear when we were on our own that if I sought legal advice, he would take me down for every cent. This was too frightening for me and so I gave Richard everything he wanted. I made the decision to stay on his good side, fearing that if I did otherwise, I wouldn't have access to my children, my family home or the dog. By doing everything Richard's way I was allowed a key to the house and to come and go whenever I pleased.

Around this time, I was seeing a counsellor and I was advised to withdraw a small sum of money from an ATM. Because Richard had never allowed me to have my own bank account, I didn't know how to use an ATM. I was finally given some help for this, but I was so frightened how Richard would react when he saw the withdrawal that it caused me severe anxiety.

Richard was absolutely furious with rage and anger. I felt very distressed!

I had fallen into a form of depression and I lacked motivation. For example, I needed flyscreens for the front and the back doors of the new townhouse. There was nothing left in my spirit to even think about ordering these, so my mother literally dragged me around Mitchell, an industrial area of Gungahlin, to get what was needed. Mum rang my father, who was living down the coast, to see if he would go halves in the cost but Dad refused. At this later stage of his life, he had changed from the generous father I knew from my childhood into being very tight with money. Due to his alcohol issues and the impact of his decisions, Dad had experienced significant financial losses through many broken relationships with women. Dad was very co-dependent and couldn't be on his own. He got involved with women who had major emotional/mental issues and most of them used him for financial gain.

Mum would often come out and stay with me in Amaroo, doing her best to try to pull me through this emotionally devastating chapter of my life. She was in a good relationship with her partner Olek, and she still chose to be there for me and support me as best she could. Mum would be smoking in my garage with the roller door up. There were so many people coming and going around us and she would often comment, "You will never feel lonely here." I know she was trying hard to pull me through and I know she had a broken heart watching me struggle to survive.

Looking back on this horrendous time of my life I have my mother to thank for staying strong and encouraging me all the way! She truly was a tower of strength and never gave up on me. I don't know where I would be today without her strong and constant unconditional love for me. Meanwhile, I would often be in tears, especially when I was out and about and I would see couples, because this made me feel I had lost everything.

However, God was looking after me because the young Catholic priest I had been seeing was building a church called Holy Spirit Parish in Nicholls, Gungahlin. I felt really blessed that I was able to go to his weekday and charismatic Catholic services. My spiritual faith kept me going during this time and, together with having full access to the family home, this greatly helped my emotional wellbeing.

Even so, this was such a hugely difficult time for me. One bright spot, which I was blessed and excited by, was Matthew and his friend Robert having dinner with me once a week. I used to get great satisfaction from buying things they loved to eat such as little meringues. Neither of my boys was sleeping at Amaroo and I was feeling desperate to have some quality time with them. I felt grateful that Matthew took the time on a regular basis to come and see me.

I also spent time planning what meals I could cook to take across to Richard and the boys. I purchased the ingredients for meals such as spaghetti bolognaise and beef stroganoff at the only Woolworths in Gungahlin and took them across to my family. This was one of the main ways I kept my sanity in the early days in my new home in Amaroo. Four out of the seven days were spent at Kaleen, being with the family and sleeping in the marital bed with Richard. He seemed very happy that I was there but after four days he would be getting agitated and wanting a break from me. At one stage he called me "one big illness". I used to come back to Amaroo absolutely drained and would often fall asleep from sheer physical and emotional exhaustion.

After two years of doing this, I woke up one morning and realised I could not continue in this way. Two years of going to the family home was making me emotionally unwell, because I was doing all the giving but getting nothing in return. For example, Richard had accompanied me to a luncheon for the chronic pain support group and there was a concert performance by the Four Kinsmen advertised. We had enjoyed seeing them in a concert at the Gold Coast in our better years and this was to be one of their last performances because they were breaking up. I wanted to book tickets, but Richard would not commit to coming, saying that we couldn't go because we wouldn't know how we would be feeling. Things like this made me feel as though Richard was having his cake and eating it too because he was enjoying all the benefits of married life without the commitment.

So, after two years, I'd had enough. It was Matthew's seventeenth birthday and I was pleased I had slept over in Kaleen and could wish him a happy birthday before he went to school. My chronic pain support group was meeting that day at Weston and I drove there and back. I was crying because it was Matthew's birthday and I knew that, emotionally, I couldn't come back to Kaleen to sleep with Richard. I simply said to the Lord, "I cannot do this anymore!" and headed straight home to Amaroo. I was distraught and crying my eyes out. This was a very hard time for me, and I was feeling so low that I called the mental health crisis team for someone to come in and see me. They were able to support and counsel me, but this was the beginning of a very long process.

Chapter 10

Going it Alone

I visited the boys regularly, sleeping in one of their beds whenever I went back to Kaleen. I continued to contribute for them financially and I was emotionally involved with trying to understand where both my children were coming from. One of these occasions was around the time of my father-in-law's seventieth birthday party. I loved my father-in-law very much. Matthew and I attended his party without Richard, who said he had a headache. Chris didn't go either, as he'd been invited to an eighteenth birthday for one of his best friends, held across the road from St Joseph's Primary School. I felt uncomfortable in my spirit about what Chris and his friends might get up to. Because both Richard's father and mine were functioning alcoholics I was worried about my boys as alcoholism ran in both sides of our family. My beautiful mother-in-law, who was always so kind to me, was also at the party. At the time, she was recuperating from a brain aneurysm. Even though physically she looked a picture of health, emotionally she was struggling, and I was concerned about her as she was saying how she just wanted to go home to be with Jesus. She had become a committed Christian not long after Richard's conversion to Christ. Richard adored his mother and they were extremely close, sharing their faith and an interest in rugby league football. He was absolutely devastated when she passed away from a second brain aneurysm two years after her first.

Driving home from my father-in-law's party, I was still uneasy about Chris and so I decided to quickly call past and check up on where he was. I saw a white van driving around in the carpark, and I assumed this was for security around the school. I couldn't hear any noise and there seemed to be nothing to be concerned about, which eased my mind. I didn't know Chris and two of his friends had trashed St Joseph's, smashing some windows. I got a call from the Principal to bring Chris in. He had been discovered as someone had recognised him as a former student of the school. The Principal was an ex-policeman—a firm man, and very wise. He cautioned Chris that this was the start of a downhill road and that he could go one of two ways. He advised Chris to think about which way he wanted his life to go.

Richard and I discussed how Chris should be punished and we decided that he must pay for the vandalization he was responsible for. We made Chris withdraw every cent from his bank account, which amounted to around $1000, and this covered the cost to repair the damage his actions had caused. Without Richard's knowledge, I also suggested to Chris that it might be a good idea for him to get away from Kaleen—and the marijuana and alcohol—for a while. He could stay at Maree's for three weeks to a month and still be able to see Linda and his friends but if he was out of Kaleen, especially after school, there was less chance to be tempted by peer group pressure. I advised Chris—without anger or shame—to use the time he was away to have a good long think about his life and to decide for himself the direction he wanted to go. I was trying to be his friend as well as his mother, and to get him out of the troubled environment he was in.

Chris decided to take my advice and so he went and stayed at Maree's. Every afternoon after school he would sit under her pergola, smoking and thinking about what to do about his life. After three weeks he came back to us a changed person. He had been deep in thought about the direction his life was to go in. Even though he was still smoking cigarettes and drinking, he was totally off marijuana—which had been the cause of his loss of motivation. By quitting it, he was able to go into Year 11 with a clear head and mind, with renewed motivation and willingness to apply himself to his school work.

Even though I was very much a part of my boys' lives, I was extremely lonely and struggling emotionally in Amaroo. Once a week, on a Friday, my loneliness was eased when my mother, four of her sisters and Maree all came to my townhouse to share lunch and participate in an Alpha course. Alpha is a series of sessions exploring the Christian faith and designed to create conversation around this. I had a strong faith and was very motivated as a new Christian to share this. Mum was not that interested, but she would still come along. I wanted to bring in the young priest to help Mum and her sisters, a couple of whom were still practising Catholics, through the course. My chronic pain group on a Wednesday and my Tuesday caring and sharing prayer group also helped keep me going.

I found it very daunting to go from being married at nineteen and then suddenly finding myself out on my own at forty-two. As a diversion from my loneliness I used to pop down to a little club called Gungahlin Lakes, which had live music. To avoid listening to the music on my own and feeling like a pick-up, I would sit at a poker machine, spend $20 or so, have a drink of champagne and be among people. I found it nice to sit and see the same people, even though I didn't know them. This gave me a sense of not feeling so alone and was my way of coping after returning from Kaleen each week.

Another place where there was live music was the George Harcourt Inn, which was a replica of an English pub. I had lost touch with a lot of my girlfriends from the past but now and again the odd single female friend and I would go there. I felt as though I was on another planet, especially because the sexual connotations in the dancing were so foreign to me.

Around the time of my birthday, I wanted to have a holiday at Murramarang Resort, which was a beautiful place with kangaroos and wildlife. The terrain was flat there, which was important for me as I was not good on my legs and I had to be careful of what shoes I wore. I paid for Maree, Matthew and one of his friends and Chris and Linda (who drove down in Chris's little Holden Gemini) to all stay together in some lovely cabins. I remember trying to get Richard to come down to the resort with us and I felt disappointed when he wouldn't. I took this to mean that he just didn't see my birthday, me or the family as a priority.

As time went by, I was having less and less to do with Richard and the more he saw I was able to cope without him, the more depressed he became. With his purpose to win compensation for me now accomplished, he was going downhill emotionally. Chris had moved out of home to live with some mates, but Matthew was still living with Richard. At seventeen, Matthew's home environment—with a depressed and unmotivated father—was very difficult. From the time he was fifteen, Matthew had put his energy into positive things such as boxing and working out at the Police Boys Club. Matthew was doing much better at this age than Chris had done. It was a huge relief to me that there was no underage drinking or smoking to deal with. I would try to think of good things to take Matthew to as I wanted to give my son an emotional lift and show him that life was still fun. I was probably at my wits end emotionally but I wanted to keep hope alive for him.

One of my girlfriends—a Christian I had met at a church service—wanted me to go on a short-term cruise sampler aboard the *Norwegian Star*. I decided this was just what Matthew needed. I also took one of his friends along. Because Richard was spending a lot of time in bed and was unable to commit to the drive to Sydney to connect with the cruise ship, I asked my brother-in-law Laurie to do this instead. I paid for the petrol and all the food along the way. Laurie dropped us off at the pier and even though I wasn't walking too well we managed to board the ship without any mishaps. We had a lovely few days on the cruise and when the time came to get off the ship and return home, another friend, Lyn, picked us up from the pier.

Lyn, whom I had known since 1994, before I separated from Richard, was one of my dearest friends. I had first met her when I attended a Christian retreat, the Golden Grove Healing Retreat at Newtown. I would regularly attend this retreat and go to all the different workshops they had—for example, on grief. Lyn had been diagnosed with a rare form of blood cancer at the same time I was diagnosed with dystonia. There was no known cure or treatment for either of our conditions. We were both desperately seeking something at the time—God? Healing? Walking through the door of the retreat, we introduced ourselves and I put my arm through hers. Lyn was an introvert and I was an extrovert and we hit it off straight away. We got on well, becoming the best of friends—and we have remained so to this day.

Lyn was willing to drive us from the pier to Sutton Forest and then Richard picked us up from there, meeting us at McDonald's. This was a big deal for someone who suffered as badly from depression and anxiety as he did, and we were very appreciative and grateful that Richard had been able to get out of the house to do this. Lyn and her husband John and their children allowed me to come to their home for extended periods of time after my marriage broke up. We loved each other's children and were able to celebrate their milestones as they were achieved.

Even though Lyn was only five years older than me, she was nurturing and loving and I used to feel emotionally safe with her. I would jump in the car to go to her place at Campbelltown and feel welcome there. I would be so emotionally exhausted from what I was going through that I would often fall asleep on one of her kids' beds. Lyn also stayed with me at Amaroo on a few occasions, which helped ease the loneliness and loss I felt through not living with my family.

I also often stayed at my dad's house down the coast. He lived with his partner and he loved me visiting. It was wonderful to stay there, and I would often go out at 11.00 am to an internet café or the movies and then come back at 5.00 pm. Dad lived in a complex of ten townhouses and all his neighbours were friendly. They would often plead with me to stay longer but Dad would tell them I was, "going back to save a sinking ship"—meaning my situation with Richard. Even though I was not living in the family home, I still felt emotionally responsible for how everyone was managing. Dad would often say to me, "Sunny, every shearer shears his own sheep," which was his way of trying to get me to look after myself.

These were very special times staying with my father as he was really getting to know me away from my sister's shadow. I do believe this was a time of real healing, because my father no longer favoured my sister over me. For the last ten years of his life our relationship had grown to the point that we were very close emotionally.

My visits to Dad's and to Lyn's gave me a little break away and some respite from Richard's depression and the intense loneliness. They were safe places where I felt comfortable. I wasn't well enough to work, and I was still experiencing gait problems and hemifacial spasms in my throat and neck from dystonia. The loss of my health, and Richard's depression, had changed my way of thinking. I now realised life was short and how important it was to be an encouragement for my children.

Chris was working hard doing his HSC and we received a phone call from Lake Ginninderra College to say he would be receiving an award at the Canberra Theatre. Richard and I went together, and we were so proud and excited when it was announced that Chris was receiving an award in every subject for being the most gifted and talented student. He decided he wasn't going on to university because he preferred working outside and so chose to undertake an electrical apprenticeship.

Chris secured a place to do his four-year apprenticeship with Electro Group, who only took the students excelling in Maths. Chris studied for hours and worked very hard, applying himself so well that he received Apprentice of the Year.

Both the sides of our families got together to celebrate Chris's twenty-first birthday, and Richard and I attended together. It was so wonderful to have everyone! At the end of the night we were driving home and Chris and Linda asked to be dropped off in the city so they could continue on, but my father, who was a big kid at heart and liked to continue to party on, jumped out of the car with them. The alcohol and partying style of life was an enormous factor in my father's life. Chris and Linda had a terrible time as they ended up at the Dickson Tradies Club listening to my father wallowing in self-pity for the remainder of the night until the early hours of the morning.

I was staying overnight at Kaleen, sleeping in Chris's room. As we were driving home, I was concerned for Richard because he thought he got caught by a speed camera. Unable to stop thinking about this, he disappeared the next day and was wandering up and down Northbourne Ave to try and work out where he was caught on camera. Richard was sweating profusely and very distressed. Even though I tried my best to reassure him that it didn't matter, and he should just wait for something to come in the mail, nothing I could say would stop his bizarre and obsessive behaviour. It was as though he was suffering from obsessive compulsive behaviour disorder. It was distressing to witness, and I felt quite bewildered as to how to help calm Richard down.

Days and weeks went past, and nothing came in the mail. I didn't realise it at the time, but this obsession was a sure sign of how emotionally unwell Richard was at this stage.

Chapter 11
Suddenly Seeking Susan

Bizarre behaviours were starting to occur more frequently with Richard and I always attributed these to stress. One particularly disturbing incident involving a keepsake from his mother caused me to realise there was much more to Richard's behaviour than just stress.

Richard asked me what I would like from his mother's things. There was a lovely purple vase which I felt would be the ideal keepsake for me. Richard's response was that he had organised a collector in to value a few things and that, instead of giving the vase to me, he could get $50 for it. I didn't feel upset or surprised as I knew he wasn't well.

Imagine my shock and distress when, months later, I came home to my place in Amaroo, only to find the vase, in a flimsy plastic bag, left dangling on an outside door handle with a note saying, "Mum would have wanted you to have it." It was a windy day, and the fragile vase could so easily have been broken. I was shocked to find it just left like that! To this day, I still have this priceless purple vase to treasure.

Other disturbing things were occurring which were very distressing for me and which made it very difficult for me to function normally. For instance, Richard would bring our beloved dog Nelson out with his food and water and tell me that I could have him, because he was saying his goodbyes. Poor Nelson stayed with me for a few days until things changed again. To be honest, I was so lonely and so broken myself it was a real comfort having him sleep on my bed with me. I enjoyed having life around me in my little place in Amaroo.

While being very distressed by Richard's bizarre behaviour, I was able to find some relief in the fact that both my boys were moving forward positively in their lives. Chris was in the third year of his apprenticeship and he wanted to get into the property market. He would ring me about a few properties he had seen, and he was particularly keen on a small townhouse in Amaroo, not far from my townhouse. He and Linda wanted to buy the townhouse together, but Linda wanted to be married before she moved in with Chris. I was able to help Chris to put in a bid and secure this lovely property. We spoke to a mortgage broker and, because neither Chris nor Linda had enough savings, I was able to lend Chris the amount of money he needed to qualify for a bank loan. He later paid me back in full without having to pay interest. I was fortunate enough to be able to help Chris because I had been left a substantial amount of money in my uncle's will—and it was such a relief to me that Chris was able to get into the property market. Renting out two of the bedrooms to two of his friends helped Chris service the bank loan. I think that moving into his own place was a good thing in that it allowed him to get away from Richard's ongoing depression. Chris loved and adored his father so much, continuing to visit the family home and seeking his advice on anything and everything he needed to know.

Matthew was also moving forward with his life, having finished his HSC year and deciding he wanted to do a double Economics degree. His home situation was becoming increasingly difficult to cope with and so he was spending more time with me at Amaroo. When Richard was unable to get out of bed for five days straight, Matthew could no longer cope, and he came to live with me. I was able to provide him with his own room at my place because I had a built-in work-station with a computer. Matthew continued to sleep between Amaroo and the family home at Kaleen. I also shared my home with another lady who had been with me long before Matthew moved in. She was company for me, helping me to ease my loneliness and cope emotionally.

Once Matthew had moved in and was legally old enough to partake in drinking alcohol, I could see that he was having problems. Once he started drinking, he did not know when to stop. He couldn't have just one or two drinks and would be wandering around after getting lost and being unable to find the friends he was out with.

I found this a very testing and difficult time, but I knew I just had to stay connected emotionally and be strong for his sake. I think I had endured so much anger from listening to my mother berate my father when he was drinking, and I did not want to react the same way with Matthew. I always left a light on and the door unlocked just to make it easier for him to let himself inside in the early hours of the morning after a night out. No matter what state he was in, I never wanted him to feel as though he couldn't come home. If he was able to come home, then I knew he was safe! My hope was that this was a stage that a lot of teenagers go through. Sadly, this behaviour with alcohol was just starting and I was going to have to endure it and try and keep my son safe for years to come.

I knew Matthew needed some emotional relief after an intense year of studying for his HSC and I was able to talk to him about this, suggesting that he take some time off to work and travel. He went ahead and joined the Public Service, getting a job in the Department of Defence. Matthew liked the people he worked with, but his job was not going to be a long-term thing. He was able to save enough money to pay for a five-week Contiki tour of the UK and Europe and, aged nineteen, went to London on his own to connect with the group of strangers he would be travelling with.

He didn't want any of my help with his packing and I knew he was feeling frustrated and needed a break from the turmoil our marriage was in. I remember feeling quite distressed by the situation, but I couldn't blame Matthew. I knew he loved us both, but our family situation was just so difficult, and it was a relief to see him going. As a mother I was very concerned for Matthew, but my faith and belief that God would take care of him sustained me at this time. Both Richard and I went to see him off at the airport. It was such an emotional time for me, because I knew my beautiful young son was hurting from all the distress and grief he had suffered since the age of eight, when I had first become unwell. The distress had been compounded by living with his father's depression and anxiety. There are no words I could write which would adequately express what Matthew went through, listening to the torment of his unwell father. As for me, I was just trying to rise above the situation and maintain Amaroo as a place of peace and comfort for Matthew when he was with me.

Matthew arrived in London but unfortunately his luggage did not arrive with him. I knew what he had in his backpack and that he was lacking in all the essentials. I followed Matthew's travel itinerary the whole time he was away, ringing constantly, trying to track his luggage. Finally, a week into the tour, I caught up with it in Monte Carlo. I tried to explain over the phone that Matthew was about to arrive and would need his luggage, but the people on the other end didn't speak English. I didn't know how Matthew was coping without his belongings, but it breaks my heart to think of him for that whole first week using the one and only jacket from his backpack as a towel to dry himself. These circumstances were all out of my control and I felt in a very powerless place, compounded by knowing that Matthew would also be hitting the alcohol hard during the tour.

My distress levels soared when, upon buying a newspaper one morning, I was confronted by a photo of Matthew and some other young people on a boat in Venice, accompanied by headlines announcing the death of an Australian boy on another Contiki tour. He had passed away after contracting meningococcal disease and, as a result, other Australians on tour had been quarantined. Alone and distraught to see my son's photo on the front page of the newspaper, I realised I couldn't do anything to help him except to put my faith and trust in God. Usually, this type of situation would cause me to be totally stressed out, but I trusted God to watch over and protect Matthew and I prayed without ceasing for the safe return of my son.

The distress I was feeling while Matthew was away was also heightened by other personal struggles I was having. I was desperate for a break from everything and for an opportunity to refresh myself and recharge my batteries. A coffee date with my friend Maria, who was also going through some trying circumstances of her own, resulted in our visiting a travel agent and booking a three-week Trafalgar tour of Europe and the United Kingdom. Within three weeks, and after Matthew's return from his trip, we were away! I had always wanted to go to Europe and the tour was just the tonic I needed.

Upon reaching Italy, the first person I rang was Richard. Unfortunately, he was so distressed by me being on the tour that he was crying non-stop over the telephone. As a reaction and accusing me of believing I was nineteen years old again, he changed his will, cutting me out of our family home we had built together, and leaving everything to our sons. I was so worn down by all that I had been through with Richard that I honestly didn't care that he had done this. His behaviour towards me was so irrational that I knew that nothing I did would ever be able to make him happy.

I didn't allow Richard's behaviour to bring me down, and even though I struggled with my mobility and couldn't do a lot of the excursions, I had the trip of a lifetime! I had learned to make the best of everything, and I was happier than many of the physically well people on our tour who always found something to complain about. Often, I wasn't fast enough to get back on the tour bus, and the Americans nicknamed me, *Suddenly seeking Susan*, which we all had a laugh about. Maria was an amazing travel companion and she helped me out whenever she could. We returned home with a deeper and richer friendship for doing this trip together.

I realised while I was away that, after all we had endured as a family, Matthew and I needed our privacy and to have time to ourselves and so I kindly asked the friend who had been sharing my Amaroo home to leave. It was a comfort to me that Chris was close by, settled in his townhouse with his friends and busy doing his electrical trade. Matthew still had time before he embarked on his double Economics degree and we had a conversation about whether he resented me for advising him to wait until he was a little older before embarking on his degree. I was relieved to find that he was pleased he had this time away from study. I had seen so many university students embark on a degree straight out of school, only to find out it wasn't right for them at all.

Matthew had also been talking to me about a young Mexican girl he had met while in Italy on the Contiki tour. My suggestion was that he should not allow distance to stop him from finding love. I knew that this came from my experience with my Sydney boyfriend when I lived in Canberra and how the breakdown of my parents' marriage had damaged me emotionally and left me unable to express my true feelings. I wanted so much more for both of my sons and so I was available to listen, with my heart, to their feelings.

Matthew decided to see if this new relationship was something worth pursuing. With my blessings and financial support, he travelled to Mexico and boarded there with an older female friend of his girlfriend's family. We didn't hear from him over the next three months, but I was at peace with this, knowing he needed this time to work through his feelings for this girl, as well as continue to get a much-needed break from Richard and me. Richard's behaviour was increasingly more bizarre and distressing. It was about to take an especially heartbreaking turn—and to go in a direction I could never have anticipated and for which I was totally unprepared.

Chapter 12

Humpty Dumpty

After Matthew's return, he and other family members, along with Richard, Chris and I, had a meal at the Gungahlin Lakes Club. Everyone was busy talking, eating and drinking. I noticed Richard hadn't finished his beer. Not wanting to appear rude, I stayed back to keep him company after the others had left. What I was about to hear filled me with a sense of overwhelming anguish and distress, the like of which I had never experienced and for which I was totally unprepared.

I cannot even begin to adequately express the crushing range of emotions I experienced when I learned what Richard had planned. Completely frozen with shock and horror, I listened to Richard inform me, in detail, of his intention to take his own life. The only details he wouldn't share with me were when or how this was going to happen. He had made up his mind he was going to go through with what he had decided was the only course of action available to him. An overwhelming sense of anxiety engulfed me and I shook uncontrollably as I tried to process what I was hearing. This was the husband I had married and the father of my children and the thought of him planning his own suicide was utterly unbearable and completely devastating.

I was so distressed by what Richard had told me that, unbeknown to him, I followed him to our family home. I needed to know he was going straight home and wasn't going to self-harm. I was on high alert and I don't believe I'd recovered from knowing he intended to take his own life. I was trying everything and anything to stay together. I didn't want to return to live in our family home because I had adjusted to central heating and a northerly aspect with my Amaroo property. My health issues needed the warmth and Kaleen was cold. Because Richard was worried about every cent, he wouldn't allow Kaleen to be heated in the way I needed it to be.

I thought if we were to sell both the family home and my townhouse we could then afford something bigger with central heating. I had found something nice and Richard and I both signed our properties up to a real estate to sell. We had looked at this home together in Amaroo and both Chris and Matthew had also looked through it. I was very keen to buy it and be under the same roof as Richard, despite being unsure how this arrangement would go after so much damage to our relationship. Feeling desperate and overwhelmed, I thought this was the only way to save Richard from going through with his intended plan. I had looked through this lovely home thirteen times and it was a nice size to give both Richard and me plenty of space to ourselves. We talked about taking walks together as the terrain was lovely and flat and nicely situated near some beautiful ponds and wildlife. It gave me so much hope.

I had also talked Richard into coming via train to the Christian retreat centre I loved to visit up in Sydney, where I had met my dear friend Lyn. It was a miracle to be able to persuade Richard to attend this and we were there for ten days. Richard cried a lot and it was difficult to gauge his mental condition. I wasn't used to this intense emotional distress and to be honest I felt out of my depth trying to cope.

When we returned home, I continued to keep myself afloat by attending my chronic pain group on Wednesdays. On one of these days I was having coffee with my friends when Richard phoned, crying and saying he was too depressed to go ahead with the sale of our family home. This was distressing because the *For Sale* signs were already posted at both our homes. The contract had been signed over to the real estate to start marketing them both.

I burst into tears as I hung up on Richard. Unable to cope with this news, I immediately jumped in my car and drove down to my father's home at the South Coast. Fortunately, the Real Estate people visited Richard and could clearly see he wasn't well. Even though there are usually consequences for signing a contract of sale and then pulling out, they were extremely understanding of our situation and I was very grateful that they decided not to take any action against us.

Our lives continued as before, with Richard constantly crying and talking about taking his life and me regularly seeking counselling. I couldn't visit the family home as often as I wanted to due to frequently feeling anxious from his threats of self-harm. I was only just holding it together myself.

Chris and Matthew were also feeling desperate to give some sort of comfort to their father and decided to buy him a newly released DVD player as he loved movies. I do feel Richard's decision for us to separate caused enormous repercussions and complications. I believe we could have worked things out more easily by staying and living within the marriage, especially as we were both committed Christians. At one stage I wanted to help a family from my church who were in dire straits and allow them to live in my townhouse. Naturally, I thought Richard would allow me to come back to the family home for a short time but when I told him of their plight and my idea to help them, his words were, "Definitely not!" I couldn't believe what I was hearing, as all this time I thought we could get back together and make our marriage work. I was totally in denial.

Matthew was still spending a lot of time in Amaroo and wanting his girlfriend to come to Australia. It was becoming increasingly difficult to obtain a three-month visa, so I decided to make an appointment with a local Member of Parliament to see if I could change the situation. I argued that if Mexico can welcome and allow my son into their country, why can't Australia do the same for his girlfriend?

As was the case many years earlier when I took on the Catholic Church, I wasn't going to back down on this issue. A long fight ensued but finally, Australia gave permission for the visa to be granted.

I realised I had a strong sense of social justice and fairness because even if the situation appeared impossible, I wouldn't let things rest until I had exhausted every avenue. I was a very strong-willed child with a lot of determination to do my utmost to make sure everyone got a fair go. I don't think this is a bad character trait when the intentions of the heart are for good. I believe I was blessed with a natural ability to advocate and persevere for others but sadly, I didn't have the awareness of my own needs.

When the day came for Matthew to be able to go up to Sydney to meet his girlfriend, I was relieved and excited for them both! After he had met her plane, both were catching a bus back to Canberra. I rang Richard to tell him, offering to pick him up so we could both go to meet Matthew and his girlfriend together. Richard declined, using the excuse that he had a few months to meet her. I was upset with him, saying he needed to do this for his son. Richard finally agreed to come but then he turned up in his slippers. At this stage, I don't think I really understood the full extent of Richard's health issues. I was just trying my hardest to do everything to hold things together.

I was relieved to finally meet Matthew's girlfriend and she was just lovely—so kind and with an understanding that life was full of joy as well as sorrow. Over the couple of months that she lived with Matthew and me in Amaroo I grew to really enjoy her company and our long deep and meaningful talks. I also loved the fact that they were regular visitors to our family home. Richard grew to really like Matthew's girlfriend. She was so humble and kind to Richard and she was very attached to the both of us.

This was a lovely time in my life but it soon came time for Matthew's girlfriend to return to Mexico. I had grown so attached to her that when it was time for her to go, I was heartbroken. I had never had a daughter and she was such a caring and loving young lady that it eased the heartache and pain of my life and gave it a real lift.

Matthew and his girlfriend continued to email and talk every day and it was wonderful that he had the opportunity to go across to Mexico and she was able to have a few months in Australia living with us. I don't really know the details of what happened between them, but I think their youth and the long-distance nature of their relationship came between them. Matthew is a very private person and never told me the details of what caused them to break up.

During the time that Matthew and his girlfriend stayed with me, Richard didn't contribute emotionally, physically or financially to help me. On several occasions, he rang up very distressed. I mentioned to Matthew that I had to get across to Kaleen to sort his father out as he was inconsolable.

Matthew's reply of, "Well, good luck, because the only person who can help Dad out is himself" was an epiphany to me! The words resonated inside me, and I needed to hear them and fully take them in. For the first time, I realised that I had no control over any of Richard's actions. I went to Kaleen and found him sobbing uncontrollably, sitting among a pile of photographs of us as a young family. Seeing him like this left me bewildered and in despair because I knew there was nothing I could do. Matthew was kind and caring with his words and wasn't saying anything to hurt his father or me.

Already numb from the countless heartbreaking conversations over the phone and the continual talk of suicide, I felt helpless because he was the father of my children. I seemed to be going around and around in circles trying to save the marriage and this was such a serious issue that I sought ongoing counselling in order to cope. The counsellor was trying to help me through and one of the things she said to me resonated with me deep within my spirit; "What you are seeking from Richard is like going to a light pole."

I was drowning emotionally with him. Nothing was working because Richard was so unwell, and I realised that nothing I said or did made any difference to him.

During this time in my life I was attending a Catholic Church and I would meet afterwards with a group of likeminded people for coffee and fellowship. I made some wonderful friends and to this day we are all in contact and help each other out whenever we can. My sister asked me to have one of her friends live with me until she found a new home, as she had sold her former home and was downsizing. I knew the friend quite well and had a lot of respect for her. I also knew she was genuine, and I wanted to help. Because of this, and with Matthew also already knowing her, I agreed to let her stay with us.

I also loved real estate, so it was a pleasure going around on weekends looking to find her a suitable home. We grew very close during this time and it was a relief to have her in my life. She was older and wiser than me and we could bounce ideas off each other, which was very good for my emotional health.

One day, we were in the car driving and as usual I was talking about Richard and how we could get back together. Her reaction was such that I knew it was too much for her to take in or deal with. It was as though everyone who was close to me and knew about my situation also knew it would never work out with Richard. It was too much for them to hear me talking about it all the time.

Trying to get back together with Richard was as impossible as putting Humpty Dumpty together again. Everything had fractured and it was insane behaviour to think I could do this, because I had tried time and time again yet nothing I said or did made any difference.

Finally, a few days before Christmas of 2003, Richard was admitted to the Psychiatric Ward in Calvary Hospital with the devastating news that he had been overusing/abusing prescription medications. Chris, Matthew and I had known nothing of this abuse. I had always put the irrational behaviour and false accusations down to extreme stress but now it was revealed just how sick Richard was. To see my husband—who had never abused alcohol and who always appeared so grounded and stable in his youth—hallucinating and delirious almost sent me right over the edge. I realised how unwell he was when he was explaining in detail how Matthew had broken into our family home with a baseball bat and had stolen some money.

Richard's conversation was all over the place and I knew that none of what he said was true. This was, without a doubt, one of the saddest times of my life. I didn't know the sadness and grief were leading me towards the beginning of a journey of self-awareness and emotional healing that was about to change my life forever.

Chapter 13

Courage to Change

I was on my way to the hospital when a friend handed me a book called *Courage to Change,* and advised me to go to a meeting called Al-Anon, which was a 12-step recovery program for people who had a problem drinker in their family. In a state of severe anxiety, I stood at the biggest crossroads of my life, having to decide whether to go to the hospital to visit Richard or to attend a meeting I knew nothing about. I think I decided to attend the meeting because I just needed to be anywhere with a friend and because what our family was dealing with was simply horrendous. I went into the Al-Anon meeting in shock and totally numb of all emotion. I was made to feel very welcome and I started listening to complete strangers share from the bottoms of their hearts. I had a light bulb moment listening to these amazing people because in so many ways their story was my story. They spoke about what I had felt and endured living with my father abusing alcohol and with my mother trying to control not only his behaviour but also mine and my sister's.

I listened and continued to go to meetings almost every day, learning strategies and tools to cope with my own life and behaviour. I couldn't get enough of it, even though I found it emotionally painful. I wished that I had been able to be in this program when I was a little girl and I would have made better decisions for my own life. Desperate and alone, I screamed out to God, "Why wasn't I here years ago?" and heard that quiet, still voice reply, "At least you are here now!"

The program provided life skills with a focus on my own self, instead of on everybody else. It was a time of great healing as my self-awareness and understanding of who I was blossomed. I realised I was a people pleaser and didn't have the ability to say no. I was also a scapegoat in my alcoholic dysfunctional family and was taking the blame for many things that were not my responsibility—for example, my sister's pregnancy out of wedlock and my father blaming me for this. I was also able to realise that it wasn't my fault that I got sick and I could apply the tools of the program to so many issues that I couldn't comprehend or didn't understand in my marriage to Richard. All his accusations—running to my local doctor, priest, family and friends, accusing and gossiping about me—I could now see as insane behaviour. I realised I didn't have to justify myself to anyone and I had plenty of character defects myself to work on. I now believed in God and could see how both Richard and I were good decent people who both came from alcoholic fathers.

Our parents were not able to nurture us in the right ways because they came from their own brokenness. Richard's control over money was to do with his sad childhood, and my inability to say no or enter into conflict on behalf of myself was coming from a place of low self-esteem and lack of self-worth.

My faith was now stronger than ever. I now believed God knew that I needed to be in Al-Anon, and He was guiding and protecting me in every area of my life. The program I was in was the same one I had been asked to attend weekly all those years ago, in order to qualify for my voluntary work for a group of psychologists. It had made no sense then, but now I was hearing and understanding it and applying it to my own life. I was excited and wanted everyone to attend because it was giving me self-awareness. For the first time in my life, I could concentrate on what was my business and what was not. I didn't have to rescue the world, and I was learning to accept things just as they were.

I had been programmed in my childhood to always help and be responsible for everyone's happiness, and now I was learning that was not my responsibility and people have to live with the consequences of their own decisions. What a relief! I now belonged in a wonderful fellowship and had made friends who were working their own program. This was a moment-by-moment, day-by-day journey for me. Naturally, I sometimes lapsed back into my old habits and reverted to my character defects, but I now had the self-awareness to know when I was rescuing, people pleasing or enabling. I could stop and be kind to myself and let go. What a relief! God had used a friend to drag me to Al-Anon at my lowest point, to show me He (God) wanted me to look after myself. I accepted that I was totally powerless over anybody else's decisions and behaviours, including Richard's, and felt sad that he was probably treating headaches and back pain in the first instance which led to a dependency.

I realised I had absolutely no control over this, and for the first time I was feeling free! The problems were all still there, but I had a fellowship to belong to, and a program that I needed to work at. I had a sponsor who made me accountable for my behaviour and character defects. Most important of all, I had a mighty God who continued to guide me through, never leaving me or forsaking me.

Richard was really struggling in hospital, going through the withdrawals of coming off all the heavy medications that he was on. On Christmas Day Matthew visited him, lying down on the floor next to his father instead of coming to lunch at Maree's. Even though it was all still distressing, I was relieved that both he and Chris were all right and that their father was in hospital getting the help he needed.

However, after only a relatively short period, the hospital said Richard was well enough to come home. This was very alarming to me as I knew he needed to be in hospital for at least a couple of months and be really nurtured and looked after until he had a chance to fully recover.

I knew Richard had changed his private medical insurance in order to get a greater refund on prescription medication. I only found that he had taken me off our private medical insurance when I needed to use it for myself. I went to talk to Richard about the fact I had to wait several months until I was eligible to claim, and that he didn't discuss this with me. His answer was that I would need extras in a psychiatric hospital and he wanted a greater refund on his prescription medication.

I saw this as his biggest downfall, as he had given up paying for private hospital cover and could no longer qualify for a private psychiatric hospital. Across the road from the public hospital was a beautiful private facility, set up for long lengths of stays without pressure of discharge. It was run like a 5-star hotel, allowing people with depression and anxiety to be respected and treated with dignity. I was frustrated and distressed that Richard was not able to have this sort of treatment, knowing in my heart that he was not well enough to be discharged from the hospital.

I was so distressed I went to Calvary Hospital and requested to see his discharge form, and it read he was not suicidal, which I totally disagreed with. Because Richard had made one of his sisters his first point of contact I couldn't argue with the hospital. I knew this was only a bandaid treatment, and the hospital system is always keen to discharge people, because they need the beds in the public system.

Upon Richard's return home, I visited with a close friend and knew all was not right. He was walking around with towels around him and on his head and was sweating profusely. I felt angry with the hospital and very distressed to see him back home, and all alone, when he had obviously not regained his mental health. I could see he was going to slip through the mental health system but there was nothing I could say or do to fix this. This authority had been taken from me, when Richard had decided to change his will because he wasn't happy that I went to Europe.

Chris and Matthew were too young to realise their father shouldn't be home from hospital. Chris had worked hard to finish his electrical apprenticeship and was preparing to go on a trip around the world. He was renting out his townhouse so he could service his bank loan—an arrangement which gave Chris a lot of freedom to take this trip of a lifetime. I was excited for him, even though having to say goodbye to him for the next twelve months wasn't easy. Chris had grown into a responsible adult and, once again, I relied on my faith that God would keep him safe and take care of him.

My belief in God had really grown and I was more relaxed at letting my children follow their dreams. With everything I was going through—including the loss of my once brilliant physical health and the devastation of many broken dreams—I was learning I didn't have control. I wanted to encourage Chris all the way and for him to leave feeling good about his decision. Before he left, he told me that when he was saying goodbye to his father there was no emotion at all from him. This felt weird to Chris. He was used to his father crying and showing emotion, yet Richard was showing no distress at all about his son being gone for twelve months.

Even though I knew Richard wasn't in a good place, I didn't want to burden Chris with this knowledge. He couldn't do anything about the situation, and I wanted him to go in peace and take the trip he had planned and paid for. To give him comfort, I said, "Don't worry. Your father isn't well but he will be all right." I told Chris to keep his head on his shoulders because he was only twenty-four years old and this was a brave trip to do on his own. Chris has a kind disposition and likes to please. I felt he needed to do this trip for himself, to go away without feeling any responsibility to his father or me.

In March 2004, I was excited for Chris to finally be able to leave Australia for his round the world trip of a lifetime!

Matthew was at university full-time doing his double Economics degree. Because the university was very close to the family home, he found it convenient to move back in with his father. I was enjoying having the company of my friend living with me, and in between looking at real estate for a new home for her, we did a lovely trip down to the south coast. I was still very much involved with all my friends from church, enjoying a wonderful social life with them and so life was going much better. I had the opportunity to take my car all around Tasmania with a girlfriend and I also flew to Darwin with two other girlfriends, where we stayed at Youth With A Mission (YWAM) at a very low cost.

Greg, one of the musicians from our circle of friends at church, had moved to live and retire in Darwin. He was doing missionary type work up there, going into the jails with his music as well as being involved with the local Christian radio station. Greg made himself available to take us three ladies around and showed us Darwin. He was a great friend and a true gentleman to us all. Greg was a shy, quiet, humble man and as I was leaving Darwin, he asked if he could email me when I returned. I had known him for years and there was no romantic spark between us. I just saw this as a compliment.

Amaroo had now become a more homely and peaceful place and Matthew would visit regularly during the day, enjoying the company of my friend and me. She had a much older son and she was very nurturing to Matthew. Matthew would often say his father was so much happier and was doing a lot of Bible study, so I felt much more relaxed and calm. I also believed Richard was doing well because he wasn't ringing as often and when he did, we would talk freely. Even though I found it strange that during these conversations he would call me "mate", I never said anything because I believed it was because he now saw me as a friend—which was much healthier for us both.

I was busy attending my Al-Anon meetings four or five times a week. I loved these meetings so much and I had a whole new group of friends in this fellowship. We would always go for coffee and share a meal after a meeting. I bonded particularly well with a kind and compassionate friend named Jenine. This was wonderful because she was in my life on a regular basis and we would share on a deeper level. I had a self-awareness that I never thought was possible and my life was the best it had been for a very long time. I could never have foreseen how much my life was about to change and to go in a direction I could not have prepared for.

Chapter 14

Rock Bottom

The morning of Wednesday, May 26th, 2004, dawned—just as so many other days before. At around 11.15 am Matthew casually walked in—just as he had done so many other times before. He had woken up to find a note from his father saying, "Out for a bit", and to discover that his father had not returned home the night before. He seemed calm and unperturbed by this but instantly I felt panic. It was highly unusual for his father not to come home all night.

I knew something was terribly wrong. I left my friend and Matthew working on the computer and left Amaroo to search for Richard.

I felt completely overwhelmed by the realisation that Richard had probably taken his own life.

I drove straight to our family home but I knew he wouldn't be there. I drove everywhere looking for him, praying that he might just be with a friend. I honestly didn't care where he was just so long as he was alive!

I spent the day searching and, in my distress, I went to an Al-Anon meeting and shared how my husband who was suicidal hadn't come home the night before. These were the only people with whom I could share this confidential information. The day was a big blur to me with the most intense emotions of despair and anxiety and a feeling of total powerlessness. I went back to the family home and Matthew was there. He wanted me to call the hospitals. I did everything Matthew wanted and rang the hospitals but Richard wasn't admitted to any of them. I rang the police to file a missing person's report, explaining he was suicidal and that he hadn't come home the night before. I don't know how I did it, but I was able to retain some sort of composure while I answered their questions.

Matthew decided to climb up to our storage cupboard and look in a box. His father had been doing a lot of Bible study, and he'd seen him putting papers away in this box. Instead, the box was filled with goodbye letters to me, his father and the boys. On top were instructions saying to feed and water our dog, Nelson. This discovery was so traumatic that Matthew and I fell, crying and sobbing, into each other's arms. We stayed in the family home while the police searched for Richard. I could tell they knew something but they weren't giving any information away at this stage.

I rang my sister and her husband, and they came to our family home. The police arrived around the same time, and delivered the gut-wrenching news that Richard had passed away. The motor of his car was still running, and the police had found his body around 7.00 pm, hidden in scrubland in an area across the road from our suburb.

Linda, Chris's girlfriend, came running in, in total distress. I couldn't help feeling that if the motor was still running at 7.00 pm at night there could have been time to find Richard because he would have still been alive until recently.

I will never forget that night for as long as I live. It was a cold night in May three days before our 29th wedding anniversary and there I was getting things together to bring our family dog, Nelson, and Matthew ready to come back to Amaroo to sleep. It was heartbreaking and I felt totally numb from the shock and horror knowing Richard had decided to take himself off this planet and away from his two beautiful sons. My heart was aching and breaking as I said goodnight to Matthew and I went into my room sobbing my eyes out because I didn't want Matthew to hear me. No doubt he was doing the same in his room by himself.

The only comfort I had was knowing my friend was in the other room. She knew what it was like to be a widow and raise a son on her own.

I was distressed about Chris in New York all by himself. The family had decided Chris needed to know, but I was afraid I might lose Chris to the streets of New York once he heard the news. What if his distress drove him to buy alcohol?

I eventually located Chris in a youth hostel. He knew already, from Richard's sisters. We didn't talk for long because the phone got cut off.

Even though I tried to contact him in the youth hostel again, I couldn't get anyone to answer the phone.

I had no idea where Chris was and what he decided to do. We could have sent money over to him to fly him home to Australia from New York but after four days of no contact, I rang Foreign Affairs to try and find him.

It turned out he'd decided to use his around the world air ticket to get back home. How sad I felt when he went from New York to London and then changed planes back to Bangkok and then to Australia. The relief to have him back home was enormous but I was sorry he had to take all these flights to come home. He did what he thought was best but to have him missing for four days after his father had taken his life is something I could never describe. Only a mother who adored her children would comprehend the anguish I felt.

One of my nearest and dearest friends found out and she drove down from Sydney. As usual I could always rely on Lyn to put herself in my position and have deep empathy. I was relieved to be in the company of a true and real friend. When something as tragic and devastating as this happens you truly know who your friends are. Most people flee because they can't cope. Also, Richard had done a lot of damage to my name and character, because he thought and said all sorts of outlandish untruths to anyone who would listen.

Luckily, God knew my heart because I was really struggling with my mobility and health, and Richard's expectations were unrealistic. He was in denial that I was physically unwell.

I wasn't consulted about the funeral arrangements. My sister and Richard's sisters did it all with the support and help of Chris and Linda. Richard's eldest sister Kay wanted to put me in the eulogy, but because I felt like an outsider and no one had taken the time to talk, ring or comfort me, I said no. I was sorry later, as I know Richard would have wanted me to be acknowledged. His goodbye letter to me was full of love and devotion. He was asking for forgiveness for leaving and at no stage did I have any anger or unforgiveness towards him; in fact I had deep empathy and understanding. He was in excruciating pain and torment. I don't think there is enough awareness or understanding around mental health and suicide.

Another close friend didn't think twice and got on a bus to Canberra to go to the funeral with me. I was grateful that Margaret came down. She'd been a friend since I was nineteen, and she understood exactly what I was going through. I needed her by my side the day of the funeral.

Two couples visited me prior to the funeral and I saw them as real, true friends, who were in deep grief themselves. This was a very lonely and grief-stricken time of my life and no one offered to drive me to the funeral. I drove myself with Margaret. Maria, another close friend with whom I had travelled to Europe, was distressed when she realised I was driving, and she and her husband took charge and drove me to the graveside.

My father came up from the coast in shock because he had always seen Richard as the son he never had.

I have only vague memories of the funeral. I was there in body, but wasn't there in my mind, because I didn't recognise people and faces and couldn't take in what was going on around me. Apparently there was a slideshow of pictures but I hardly remember seeing it; everything was a complete blur. I remember saying to my mother that

I didn't want to go to the wake, but she insisted I go. At the graveside I can only remember struggling to balance as I threw the dirt on the grave, and saying to God, "The best thing I can do now is to stay sane for my boys."

I knew both my sons needed me more than ever, and I had to be strong even though I felt like shattered glass.

I made a brief appearance at the wake, and some people said hello and offered me their condolences, but I actually couldn't recognise them. The shock must have been so great that I don't remember the people, events and/or details to this day. I just dragged myself to the church without noticing what I wore. All I wanted to do was go back to my little place in Amaroo. Once I returned there I started to feel a little better, because I was around a couple of friends who loved me and I felt safe.

Chris moved into my place at Amaroo and slept in the lounge room, Matthew was in his own room, and my friend, who was the biggest blessing in disguise, helped us all through. It was a packed home and we had our beautiful little Nelson now living full-time in Amaroo.

Chris cleared out our family home by himself, getting it ready to go up for sale. He spent days there doing all the cupboards and personal memorabilia and he had a record of all the medication Richard took and listed it all. It was such an emotional task for someone his age, and he did everything to perfection.

There was a garage sale of all our furniture and utensils, and I will never forget that day. I went over, thinking I could help. People arrived and I knew I shouldn't have come. I knew every bit of the history of when and how we bought everything, down to plates, books and eggcups. It was distressing, and my sister, as well as Richard's side of the family, were all there.

It was as if pieces of my heart were being ripped away. To see all your furniture taken out of the home you had built when you were so young, and strangers taking everything... To be watching it all brought me probably the closest I have been to wanting to take my own life.

By the grace of God, the same friend who had given me the book *Courage to Change* was with me and wanted to get me out of there quickly. My friend took me to an Al-Anon meeting where I could sob my heart out to a room full of people who were understanding and were on the same journey of self-awareness that I was on. I know without a doubt God was in all this with me, because He knew exactly what was happening and He was protecting me. I felt much better once I did the meeting and was able to go back to my home in Amaroo with clarity of what was important and what was not.

I pulled myself together. I was a parent, and I was putting up my hand to God, saying, "I brought these two beautiful sons into the world and I am never going to be a victim or abandon them!"

Seeing my whole life's work and earnings being taken by so many strangers had pushed me to the lowest point in my life.

My mother was my rock at this stage, and she and the lovely friend living with me pulled me through. They made me get a couple of chairs that my sister was planning on taking down to her onsite caravan. My mother insisted I should have them. I was able to place them in my little Amaroo home. I had worked hard and paid for my beautiful furniture that was given or sold to strangers and it was such a blessing to have just two chairs from my Danish Deluxe collection. I will always be grateful to my mother and my friend living with me for making me stand up for myself and hold onto two pieces of my furniture for keepsakes.

My father had written me a beautiful card of love and support, expressing his concern about how on earth was I going to get over this tragedy. I felt loved and supported by some really good faithful friends and both my parents, so I kept company with only them, because I knew they had my back. I didn't want to pursue any relationships with people I didn't trust or respect.

112

The 12-step recovery program was working, and I loved getting to my meetings, because I was receiving awareness such as I had never known, and getting to know who and what was good for me.

Chapter 15

Farewell Snowy Place

Our Snowy Place home was finally sold in September 2004, and all the wonderful memories of the parties, Christmas celebrations, our neighbours, and Chris and Matthew's childhood years, were all going with this house that the boys loved so much. Matthew was only twenty-one, and he slept there by himself at night, right up until the night before the settlement date when the new owners would be receiving the keys to our family home. This is how much our family home meant to him. We weren't happy that Chris hadn't got to do his round the world trip, so when the house was sold he went back overseas to do what he started to do. It was wonderful to see him have the strength of character to keep going with his life and dreams. Matthew continued with his university degree, and I was relieved to see both the boys following their dreams. I seemed on the outside to be doing really well, and I was determined to never allow my sons to see me grieve or cave under the pressure I was feeling. I was always upbeat around them but my grief was very private. I had lovely caring friends around me and yet I felt lonely.

Greg had been emailing me since I visited Darwin and we had gotten to know each other on a deeper level. He was a great support and friend and wanted to come back to Canberra. I called him in Darwin at 3.00 am and told him that I wasn't relationship material, that I wasn't well and didn't want him coming down from Darwin for me. He loved it up there and it was his heavenly paradise. He said he'd prayed about it and would come down and get his own flat and there would be no pressure.

My mother was supporting me emotionally through so much, and I was trying to get on with some sort of life. One day my mother and I were at the Dickson shops, and I thought I was all right, but out of the blue I found myself crying in every shop and I couldn't control myself. My mother was trying to comfort me and wanting to buy me everything and anything to try and console me, but nothing was going to make any difference. I agreed to one small crystal love heart that I could put up in my home, but that was to remind me of my mother! She really was the only friend I felt loved me unconditionally. It was a distressing scene and I should not have been out in public, because the crying continued and I couldn't stop—I didn't seem to have any control. Nothing could console my deep heartache. They were such intense emotions—I don't think anyone could comprehend it including myself.

I started to journal, writing all my thoughts and feelings down, and this seemed to help take the power away from my emotions.

Matthew, my friend and I were all living together with Nelson. I wasn't very well emotionally but kept going to my Al-Anon meetings, doing at least five meetings a week to be able to share my feelings and also listen to others so I could learn how to cope. I continued to go to church with my friends and try to find some sort of normality in the loss. I had deep grief for both my sons and wanted to take their heartache and pain away, but all I could do for them was to provide a warm safe home, especially for Matthew.

Matthew was drinking alcohol a lot with his friends but was still able to continue with his degree. No doubt Chris was doing the same, but overseas where I couldn't hear or see what was going on.

The twelve months soon went by, and Chris arrived back home. He had loved his travel experience and it was a huge relief to me that he was home safely. I knew he had to make many changes, because he didn't have a job and his property was rented out, but his relationship with Linda was still really good which made me very happy. Linda had loved Richard, so Chris had Linda to share the grief and loss with. Chris was still in a lot of emotional pain. He had shared with me that he dreamed of his father all the time, and was waking up with tears running down his face, and this went on for a very long time. It was a pain I wanted to take away from him, but I couldn't. All I could do was listen and do all I could to make both my sons feel safe and secure.

Nelson our family dog was finally free from lying around in a depressed household, and it felt wonderful to give this beautiful little dog some quality of life. He was going on regular walks thanks to my friend who was living with me, because my mobility wasn't good enough to take him. I had a doggy door put in to give him his independence, and even though he was old, we taught him to go backwards and forwards through the door. I had someone come on a regular basis to wash and groom him. He was very proud of himself, and would run through my little Amaroo home with great excitement and delight every time he was washed, clipped and pampered. He was happy, and didn't have any problem adjusting to the new living arrangements, because he knew he had Matthew, Chris and me to love and care for him.

Both the boys were financially well off because Richard had left our family home to them, and once the funeral expenses and all the costs of selling our home were paid, the remainder was split between them. I thought they were very young to get such a large amount of money and hoped and prayed they used it wisely, but I felt it wasn't my business and we never discussed how they intended to spend the money.

In late November 2004, Greg arrived down from Darwin and he settled into an old but homely rental flat. He could see that I was heavily involved in the 12-step Al-Anon program and came along to some meetings with me, as well as getting involved in the music ministry at church. I was able to gather some furniture together with the help of my generous mother to help make his flat more comfortable. He was happy to help and support me and/or Matthew in any way that was practical. I was still enjoying the company of my friend living with us, and she was still trying to find the right property to buy. As far as I was concerned, there was no hurry. I believe having her with me when Richard died was providential. She made Matthew's bed every morning and would leave a little bar of chocolate as a treat for him. It was wonderful for Matthew and me to have this continued support and encouragement.

In February 2005 my friend found her own place and moved out, after we had enjoyed one another's company for fourteen months. I was really excited for her, because it was a lovely home and lifestyle she had found. I knew we were going to be friends on a deep level forever, because we had gone through the tragedy together, and Matthew had grown really attached to her as well. I felt sad because we were parting ways. I didn't want her to go, and I didn't want to tell her that, because I knew it was time.

Greg was helping in different ways, such as walking our Nelson, and at one stage I flew over to Perth to have some time away with a dear friend named Thea. I was coping quite well, but Matthew got in touch with Greg to say Nelson wasn't well and it appeared he'd had a turn of some kind. I caught the first flight home. It must have appeared bizarre behaviour to my Perth friend, but Nelson represented a close tie with Richard and the last link with him that the boys and I had. After a rush to the vet, I was told Nelson was in severe heart failure. This was the start of heart medication and giving him only short walks. Nelson often needed to be carried home while he was on a walk. We were all distressed because we couldn't make a decision about Nelson. Chris felt it was time to say goodbye to Nelson, while Matthew felt that while he was still wagging his tail and eating, we should let him be. I virtually lived at the vet's, and I was so emotional that I don't think the vet knew what to do. Nelson was now on heavy heart medication to drain the fluid that was building up around his heart, and he needed to sometimes be at the vet in crate rest. This ongoing care of Nelson was costing me a fortune, and I wasn't prepared to have him put down until Matthew was ready. I was just relieved that Nelson had at least one year of quality life, living with us in my Amaroo home, but the time was getting really close to having to say our goodbyes.

In August 2006 I was at the physiotherapist, and Nelson was at the vet in crate rest, when I received a call from the vet to say Nelson had taken a heart turn, and because my mobility was so slow and it was a long way to drive to be with Nelson, I gave permission for the vet to let Nelson go. I felt it was selfish to make this beautiful little dog stay in distress while I tried to get there.

I called Chris and Matthew, and we all went to the vet while he was still warm, to say our goodbyes. Matthew was at university, and drove in distress to get to Nelson. Chris dug a grave, and we placed Nelson in the ground—it was such an emotional time! I said a prayer with both the boys, and then Matthew needed to have a shower to release his emotions in privacy while Chris covered over the grave. Our last link with Richard had gone and the boys and I felt empty.

Greg was very kind and caring, but I didn't know what was happening to me. I thought I was coping but all of a sudden an enormous wave of severe depression would come over me. It would occur out of the blue, and I would be depressed for up to twelve hours until it lifted. On one occasion I was at a movie with Greg, and needed to go to the toilets, and an enormous panic attack came over me. I returned to the movie and didn't say anything to Greg, and I was stressed trying to get through the movie, and when it was over I had to tell Greg I needed to get back to Amaroo. The panic attack was so bad that I couldn't stay and even have a coffee with him. I was so bad that I couldn't get petrol by myself without panic. This interfered in my daily life. Greg would buy tickets to a concert, and I would get to the outside of the venue, and then panic would come over me and I couldn't stay, and ended up having to come home. I had no idea what was happening to me—the waves of depression and anxiety were horrendous, but I never told Chris or Matthew, because I wanted them to think I was well and coping.

I enrolled myself in a closed depression and anxiety course, which was a full day once a week for two months at a private hospital, to try and get help. I was very lucky that I had private hospital and medical health insurance. I was with women and men who had faced trauma, and it was hard going, as this course would trigger all sorts of emotions. In fact it was so difficult that half the people in our group ended up in hospital, because it triggered all the emotions and they had a breakdown. I am grateful that I was able to listen and work through all the projects the professionals gave us. I found out I was having intense panic attacks, anxiety and depression from the suicide, and it was not going to go away overnight. I learned that I had to stay where I was when the panic came over me, even if for five minutes, and slowly increase the time I stayed, because the more often I went straight home the less likely it was to go away.

I was relieved that the professionals running this course understood it was reactive trauma, and they felt confident that I wouldn't stay like this forever. I was given tools to implement in my everyday life. It took the best part of two years to recover, and slowly the depression and panic attacks subsided and eventually went away. It was such a relief to be able to plan outings and be able to stay in a group of people, without the panic-driven urges to rush back home. I felt grateful to the kind and caring people I had around me who helped me through these difficult two years.

Matthew was slowly recovering, and he mentioned he was going to play golf with a girl from university. I said, "Oh! that sounds nice," and asked if they were any more than friends.

He reassured me with a "No!" but I knew Matthew and he was just trying to keep it low key at this time. Eventually I was able to meet Krystal, the girl who had played golf with Matthew, and it was lovely to see them together. I knew Matthew would not allow any of his family to meet a girl unless there could be a future with her. This was the start of their relationship. I was concerned that Matthew was still drinking a lot, and his group of male friends were very important to him, because they had known Richard and had also witnessed the distress of Matthew and our family, as they were all at the funeral. This was a tight, close group of friends, and Matthew was very happy having his mates around him as there was a lot of history, so it was a great comfort to know Matthew had some amazing males to talk to about his loss. They all supported each other in many ways.

I was concerned Krystal might not have known about the loss of Richard, and there was an opportunity to have some time with her. I felt she deserved to know, because she was only nineteen, and there would be a better chance of their relationship working if she knew. I could see that she genuinely cared for him and she was very loyal, honest and faithful. It was a short but nice talk, and Krystal said she hadn't heard anything from Matthew, but his good friends had told her. They also were at university together, so it would help them both, because they were needing to spend time on their degrees for their futures. Matthew took a while but he eventually opened up to Krystal as the trust and respect grew between them.

Chris had decided to move out of Amaroo as he needed his own space, so he moved into a group house with his mates from school. On a few occasions I would struggle with my impaired mobility and take a meal down to Chris where he was living, because at that stage he wasn't working. He would talk to me a lot about having his own business, and the decision he was trying to make was between maintaining vending machines or opening a noodle shop. I listened to all the pros and cons about these types of businesses and it was good because, even though Linda was working, it would involve them both if they were to start out in business for themselves. I trusted Chris with whatever decision he would make, because he would do all the groundwork, and wouldn't leave any stone unturned in getting to know what he was going into. He loved all his talks and ideas he had with his father, and I knew this was an enormous loss for him and would continue to be for a long time. Chris was the type of person who would cross all his T's and dot all his I's, so even though it would be a risk, he would put his whole heart and soul into anything he wanted to achieve.

On a cold and rainy day in September 2005, Chris was doing the fit out of his first Wokitup noodle bar in Gungahlin. He was twenty-five and high up on a ladder when an elderly Asian man wanted to know who the owner of this shop would be. I was standing talking to Chris and heard him tell the elderly gentleman, "The owner is a lady."

He took all his details down so he could pass it on to Linda, who later employed this man as their first chef.

Chris was keeping a low profile, and even though this was a very exciting time for both him and Linda, they weren't very familiar with the food industry and what was involved. It was an enormous risk!

Luckily, they were both young, had their health, and were both willing to work hard with everything they did. Chris talked about how his father would cope if he was here to see him. We both agreed Richard would be having a nervous breakdown watching Chris take such an enormous risk, not to mention the workload this involved. Chris was good at involving me in so many details and wanting my opinion on what the name of this shop should be. I was very interested and listened to all the details, and could see both Linda and Chris would give it one hundred percent. I encouraged them both all the way, as Chris could do most of the fit out of the shop. Because he was a qualified electrician and very gifted and talented with anything he put his hands to, he was able to save quite a lot of money, which was an enormous benefit for them.

This was the most exciting time for me, not to mention all the family on our side and Linda's.

I was very nervous for Chris and Linda, especially as the big opening day was about to happen. I told everyone and anyone so they could have as much support as possible on the opening day. Wokitup Gungahlin was all ready with vibrant balloons and colours and a spectacular fit out inside this amazing shop, and the doors were opened to the public in October 2005. I couldn't have been more proud as this new innovative form of casual dining was introduced to Canberra. I was watching Chris closely, and to see him serving behind the counter was exciting and I could see he was very capable. The queues were enormous as the public waited to be served, and the woks were busy clanging, making such a sound as the chefs cooked in front for all to see these delicious meals being created.

The concept was to build your own box, which was to pick the type of noodles, sauce, vegetables and/or meat you would like—the range of meats were pork, seafood, chicken and beef, with an array of vegetables—bean shoots, carrot, broccoli, onion, bok choy, capsicum, snow peas, corn, tomatoes, peas and shallots. This was such an enormous endeavour for two twenty-five-year-olds who had no experience in this type of work, to start from scratch with no one to train them. It was enormous and very impressive, and I couldn't have felt prouder of both Chris and Linda, because they had both come from humble beginnings.

Chris and Linda had both their families and friends there to support them. Matthew was even in a photo shoot, so he was the male face of Wokitup! I wished with all my heart that Richard could have been here to see this extraordinary achievement.

My mother was so proud! She loved every minute of it all, and it was a dream come true for her and for me in many ways, because both my mother and I were very driven people in our youth, but we had married a different type of person, and this type of achievement needed two driving forces for it to become a reality and a success.

Chapter 16
Celebrating Life

In April 2006 Chris and Linda returned home from a holiday in Fiji, and Chris rang me, wanting me and anyone I could bring to come down to his shop, because he had news for us all. I was grateful my mother was now living not far from me in Amaroo, and Matthew was able to come with us.

We all congregated at the shop, and the big news was that Chris had taken Linda to Fiji and got down on bended knee and proposed to her in a beautiful swimming pool. I can't believe it came as such a shock to me, because they had dated since they were fourteen and fifteen years old. I was excited once they had convinced me that they were now engaged, and would be getting married on October 7th the same year, so this was a short engagement.

Chris rang me later and wanted me to explain to Linda why he wanted to be married in All Saints Anglican Church in Ainslie. This was very important to him because this was where he was taught Sunday School with his father as the teacher. Linda was very understanding, and so the church was booked and all the arrangements were set in motion for their wedding day.

Greg's time living in the old flat my mother and I had put together was over, as his doorways were eaten away by white ants and everything was falling around him. He had decided to buy off the plan in a complex called Carnaby, which was part of the Big W construction project in the Gungahlin Town Centre. We had seen it as a "piece of sky" above the partly built lower levels, and had thought we still don't know our future, but Greg felt keen to put a deposit on this apartment and get off the dead rent cycle. This also meant that he would be closer to us, and would have a lovely warm sunny aspect which he badly needed, as he is a chronic asthmatic. We both enjoyed watching this apartment go up slowly over a couple of years.

My mother was still living near me in a lovely home, but she suffered depression and anxiety. She came to me crying, because water restrictions were on and she couldn't cope with her front and back garden not getting enough water. Even though my mother presented as strong and very dominating and opinionated, she wasn't emotionally well. She had never learned to drive, and she loved the shops, so I said I might be able to get an apartment like the one Greg had purchased. I felt very blessed when I contacted a real estate agent and there was one available on the other side, looking straight into Chris's Wokitup store. My mother was delighted because she was finally able to enjoy her large balcony and watch the world around her, and this was the solution to her depression; not having to worry about gardening and mowing lawns.

My father was visiting from the South Coast. He was in heart failure but had a positive attitude, and his drinking days were over! He wanted to see Chris's shop, and he was so impressed! He finally had a grandson who took after him with a flair for building. He loved having a coffee with me while he watched the apartments going up in big concrete slabs. He was a retired builder, and everything had changed since his days of building in the A.C.T. He couldn't do much because of his breathlessness, but he was managing to balance his heart medication as best he could. Heart failure on my father's side of the family was genetic, and no one I knew in the family had lived past seventy-nine. My father had a partner, and it wasn't an easy relationship on either me or my sister, but we put up with it, as we knew our father couldn't cope with being alone. So long as he was happy, that was all that mattered to us as his daughters.

Chris and Linda were keeping very busy with the enormous success of their Wokitup shop as well as arranging their wedding, and we were all excited for them both. I was struggling with my mobility, and trying to find a nice dress to wear to my son's wedding, and manage in flat sandals, was very important to me. I had no idea what was happening to my mobility, and thought it was all connected to the nerve damage in the right side of my head and throat, from the reaction I had in 1991. I was still seeing my neurologist who was writing in his reports that I had Dystonia.

I was very keen to be able to do a good speech for Chris on his wedding day, and I was quite emotional, because I had to do this on behalf of Richard as well as myself. Everything was still very fresh, and I was thinking this is the first big milestone Richard and I should have been enjoying together and he wasn't here. This was the start of many a milestone I was going to have to see through alone.

Chris and Linda were very generous to me, and asked me to make a list of people who I would like to have as guests at their wedding. This was a great comfort, as I was surrounded by so many of my faithful and good friends who stayed by my side before and after Richard passed away.

On the 7th October 2006, Chris and Linda were married in front of all their family and friends, and it was wonderful to have a beautiful celebration of their love and lives. We needed a celebration after what we had all endured in 2004! I had my hair and makeup done and was in the lift returning to get dressed when all of a sudden the lift stopped with a jerk and refused to move up or down. I pushed the emergency button and had to wait for twenty minutes, which felt like a lifetime, worrying that I was going to miss Chris's wedding. Just in the nick of time the lift was released and I had to rush getting dressed.

I just had enough time to check on Chris, Matthew and one of Chris's best friends, making sure they all looked suave and sophisticated. As they were getting into a limousine, Chris asked me to hop in with them. I didn't feel confident on my legs and knew I was safer to go with Greg and Krystal, because I could lean on Greg while trying to navigate the terrain and the steps of the church.

The day was just perfect. Linda arrived in a beautiful horse-drawn carriage, and everything went to plan. I was very proud of how responsible Chris was, and knew without a doubt he would take his marriage vows seriously and make a wonderful husband to Linda. It was very important to me that they had a Christian marriage and made their vows between themselves and God.

Matthew on the other hand was still only twenty-three and drinking too much, and still very raw from the loss of his father. Even though he was going out with Krystal, he still had a lot of growing up to do. I was approached a few times during the wedding reception about Matthew's alcohol consumption, and I approached him but he wouldn't listen to me. There was nothing I could do about it, and even though it made me stressed watching him, I had enough of my Al-Anon program within me to know I was in a powerless position. I also was determined I wasn't going to allow Matthew's excessive drinking to stop me enjoying this amazing and exciting day for Chris and Linda. It was their day!

I was delighted when Chris and Linda wanted me to take them to the airport the next day to fly out to the Maldives for their honeymoon! They had involved me in every aspect of this amazing and exciting day. I had been able to go with Linda to a wedding expo, view the invitations and know all the fine details, and taking them to the airport was an honour. I had lost Richard, and here I was gaining a beautiful caring daughter-in-law to marry my son. She made me feel loved, wanted and cared for. That is all any parent ever wants, to see their children happy and in a loving relationship.

We continued on with our lives, and Matthew was working hard doing his double Economics degree. That was my main focus, living with Matthew on my own in Amaroo and making myself emotionally available for him, because I knew he had gone through so much more trauma, and witnessed and heard Richard's mental health issues the most. Even though I was extremely worried about his drinking binges, I understood that he was having his own struggles and grief with the loss of his father, and I was proud he was continuing on with his degrees. I had great confidence that if we rode this out, with great respect and unconditional love, Matthew would finish and go on to pursue his dreams. I wanted both my boys to feel they could take risks wherever their passions were, and I would support them one hundred percent.

I had always said to them both, "Nothing ventured, nothing gained." I felt secure in who they were both becoming, and knew they both had very good and kind hearts full of compassion.

Later in 2006, Matthew finally finished his double degree in Economics. It was another very exciting milestone to be present at the graduation night, and it was wonderful to have Chris there taking all the pictures. Chris and I were proud of Matthew and all the hard four years of solid studying he'd got through, especially with no break while he was grieving the loss of his father. Matthew proved what I had always known, that he was extremely bright academically, with a very analytical mind, which was obvious to me even when he was as young as three. He was also the first person from his father's and my immediate side of the family to go on to university and work hard and get a double degree. It was also very exciting, because Krystal and Matthew were in a relationship, and they both received their degrees at Parliament House on the same night! To have both my sons following their dreams, in amongst such tragedy, was beyond any words I could ever express.

Greg had moved into his lovely new apartment and was still wanting to marry me. I didn't feel like marriage material and we had discussed this at length. I was calling out to God for wisdom and a sign because we were both Christians and didn't believe in living together. I didn't want to move into his apartment and leave Matthew, and Greg was a free spirit and had had fifteen years on his own. He wasn't conventional and was happy to have a flexible marriage, which made it more attractive to me.

I had been on a few silent retreats in my Christian walk, for up to five days at a time, and on one occasion someone left a scripture under my door. It was from Isaiah 43:18,19 (NIV)—Forget the former things; do not dwell on the past. See, I am doing a new thing! Now it springs up; do you not perceive it? I am making a way in the wilderness and streams in the wasteland.

I kept this scripture close to my heart, and because there was no conversation with the other participants and I didn't know anyone, I felt this scripture was from God to me. I related to every word, because I sure had felt in the wilderness over the many years of intense struggle. I didn't want another failed marriage, and if I was to marry Greg it had to be supernatural as far as I was concerned.

Greg had spent months in prayer as to whether he should leave Darwin, and taken months to return to Canberra.

I continued to pursue God and to seek His divine will for my life, and I prayed and asked God to confirm His words for me by giving me the scripture from Isaiah 43, and this would be confirmation to go ahead with my marriage to Greg. I was driving to physiotherapy for exercises for stretching the length of my Achilles tendons, something that was difficult to stay on top of, as I had no idea why I was losing my mobility. I was listening to 1WAYFM, our local Christian radio station, and a lovely song was playing, and the lyrics in this song were the exact words from Isaiah 43:18,19. I knew without a doubt this was not coincidental and this was from my faith in God, that He was confirming this marriage between Greg and myself was of Him and not of ourselves. I felt relief and joy, but panic as well, because I didn't feel physically well enough to marry Greg.

I kept this to myself and didn't confide in Greg or anyone. I continued to call out to God, and asked Him to confirm this was definitely His will for both Greg and me, so I asked him to give me the same scripture again.

Not long after, I was rushing out, and put the keys in the ignition of the car. I was by myself in Amaroo, and a man was sharing the same scripture of how he knew he had to move forward after his business had gone into liquidation. He used Isaiah 43:18,19. I couldn't believe what I was listening to, coming from the radio station. I knew I had tested God over and over again, and He was faithful, and it was time to act on His promise to me, that He was doing a new thing, and He was making a way in the wilderness and streams in the wasteland of my life.

I was finally able to share this with Greg, and because we both shared the same faith, it was easy because he believed me. We decided to have a reasonably small wedding, and have it close to my fiftieth birthday so we could celebrate both these special occasions together.

Chris and Matthew were not keen for me to get married in a coloured dress, so I felt blessed when I was able to find a lace ivory layered dress. My sons were very accepting and happy for me, which made a tremendous difference to how Greg and I would start out as husband and wife.

There was no decision who I wanted as my maid of honour; my dearest friend Lyn was with me through so much of my suffering and loss, and I wanted her to be right there beside me on this very special day. My mother was very involved, to the point of interfering, but she was excited and pleased for me, so it was wonderful to have her acceptance and blessing. My father was so sick by this stage, it was touch and go whether he would be well enough to drive up from the South Coast, but I knew my father well, and if he could get there he would do his best. After all the loss and tragedy, he would want to be there. I asked Chris and Matthew to walk me down the aisle, and they were caring and kind to me, and accepted Greg into our family, as they had grown to really respect and like him.

On Friday the 26th January 2007, Greg and I were married in the company of our families and our friends. I had gone to a lot of trouble to invite only people who I felt genuinely loved and cared for us both. We were blessed to have the young priest who had helped me through my suffering and tragedy, and the pastor of the church we were attending, to officiate together at our marriage ceremony. It truly was a magical and exciting day! There were no second thoughts, and a peace came over me that this was God's will for both our lives.

It was Australia Day, and we were right on the lake, celebrating our wedding at the Boathouse by the Lake. The Australia Day fireworks (which we decided were put on especially for us) were just magnificent! It truly was a wonderful celebration and I was able to blow the candles out for my fiftieth birthday. This really was the start of a bright, new and happy time of my life.

We had decided I wouldn't move much across to Greg's apartment, because Matthew and I were living together, and I wanted to go between my Amaroo home and Greg's. Our homes were so close to each other that I was looking forward to having some time in my own home with Matthew. I left my bed and all the furniture and brought only some clothes across to Greg's place. We both loved Greg's brand-new apartment, and it was a very exciting time of our lives.

We had a wonderful honeymoon of six weeks away up north and did a bit of travelling from one place to the next, and we had the privilege of my girlfriend Lyn and her husband John joining us for a week. We had a wonderful relationship with them and felt so comfortable in one another's company. I was still struggling with my mobility and needed help in and out of the pools wherever we went. Greg and I weren't worried at this stage, because the battle of my mobility and neck spasms had been going on since 1991, and I thought it was part of Dystonia, so I was just living with it.

Krystal's parents had moved up north to retire, and Matthew told me she was looking for a shared home. She had her beautiful cocker spaniel called Aussie, who was an old boy with attitude, and both Matthew and Krystal truly loved and cared for him. It was making it difficult for Krystal to find a place to live when she had Aussie to bring with her. Eventually Krystal and Aussie moved into Amaroo with Matthew, and I had to find a place to store my bed and bedroom suite and many other things. I was able to leave all my solid timber furniture in my lounge room. It was all happening for Greg and me as well as for Matthew, Krystal and Aussie. We were all adjusting to very different living arrangements that none of us had planned for or foreseen and even though we all had a roof over our heads it was a big adjustment, especially for Krystal and Matthew because they weren't long out of university and they both had new employment responsibilities.

Greg and I had some wonderful years living in his Carnaby apartment and life was so much simpler. We found it freeing to be able to go out with our friends and catch a movie spontaneously, and enjoyed having no responsibilities to gardens, pets, etc. These were really tremendous years and we felt we were living the life we had both always dreamed of doing. We enjoyed our married life together because our children were grown up and getting on with their lives. I persuaded Greg to go on a few cruises with me and he loved it. We loved the dining experience, all the variety of live entertainment, not to mention Greg was always one of the first to put his name down to sing at the Rock-a-oke or Karaoke. We enjoyed all the ports of call and it was a wonderful way for us to relax and travel. Nothing was tying us down, and we could take off at short notice and stay in luxury resorts in Fiji, Cairns or wherever a whim took us. I felt grateful my health was holding up well and we were able to have some amazing cultural experiences.

We lived above all the shopping centres and great eateries, and sometimes Greg would walk down to get a few groceries, and I noticed he would return home without some of the important items. This happened a few times, and we decided to check if all was well with his health. After thorough tests over a long period of time, it came as another hurdle we were both going to have to adjust to. Greg was diagnosed with executive function deficit. Executive function includes the ability to plan, initiate, monitor and control one's activities and behaviour, regulate attention and emotions, ability to empathise with others and adapt to change. Test results showed that Greg's intellectual functioning was in the superior range of ability and in fact was in the gifted range. We were called in for an appointment, and it was explained that this was not a mental illness but it was a significant disability, and we would have to rearrange our lives around it, just as it was with my diagnosis of glossopharyngeal neuralgia and dystonic gait disorder. We had an enormous challenge on our hands, with me having to do all the initiating, organising and memorising, and Greg having to do a lot more leg work and helping me in a physical capacity. Greg and I were strong in our faith and commitment to each other, and knew that God had brought us together, and we were not going to let this deter us from having a loving and fulfilling life together.

Chapter 17

Achievement and Grief

In February 2007, Chris and Linda opened up their second Wokitup store. It was exciting to see another brand new and bigger store, and we were once again proud and present at the Grand Opening of Wokitup Belconnen. Both Chris and Linda were very busy, but young, healthy and very driven. It was a really good time of their lives, giving work opportunities to so many young people, either still in college years or at university. Chris had built another beautiful shop, once again making a big saving because he did most of the fit out himself.

Matthew had secured a position in the graduate program in Department of Treasury, and he was placed in a budgets area for a twelve month period, while Krystal was a human resources manager with the Sportsman's Warehouse. They were both successful in securing these positions because of the degrees for which they had both worked so hard. In 2008, Matthew secured a position with Proprietary Futures as a trader, and this meant he needed to live and work in Sydney. This was a big move for him, but he wanted and needed to pursue and take risks, because he had become his own person and this was a wonderful opportunity. Krystal had Aussie and needed to stay in Canberra until they could find someone to look after Aussie or find a home with a backyard in Sydney. Sydney proved a difficult place to live in, especially when you are renting and looking for an appropriate rental with a backyard that allows animals.

Once Krystal found someone honest and reliable to stay and mind Aussie, she was able to move to Sydney to join Matthew. Krystal was busy working with Swisse Wellness Pty Ltd, and she and Matthew commuted between Canberra and Sydney for a long time because they still had the responsibility of Aussie. As the time went by they found a home in Sydney with a backyard and Aussie was able to join them, so they no longer had to do that long commute. Aussie was getting old and his health was failing, but the love they had for this beautiful legend of a dog was remarkable.

Matthew was busy co-founding a hedge fund called TallShip Capital Management. He would be one of six founding partners to manage money on behalf of international clients using statistical models. Krystal was onboard a hundred percent with this very important decision, and she was the main breadwinner while TallShip was being established. This was a very exciting time for Matthew, to be following his dreams and learning important information that he would go on to use half a decade later. I felt proud of him, and it was wonderful to visit him at the TallShip offices on George Street in Sydney, the nerve centre of the operation where international commodities, foreign exchange, bonds and equity indices were being traded. To get this off the ground took countless hours, days and nights, with hardly any sleep.

Greg and I found ourselves with the decision to either live in my Amaroo home and rent his apartment, or sell up and update to a new home. We were trying to decide what to do with both properties, now that Matthew and Krystal had moved to Sydney to live. It was a difficult decision because we loved both properties. I was intending to give Amaroo a little makeover when I realised I was struggling down and back from the communal bin area with my mobility. I loved the aspect—it was on a hill with gorgeous sunny views, but I couldn't walk up the hill to collect my mail. I made a snap decision to sell it, and I was on a roll. I had it painted and the gardens manicured, and it was looking just beautiful. My mobility and balance were slowly deteriorating, and I knew I couldn't cope or manage it with the slope it was on. We had enjoyed three fabulous years in Greg's apartment, but the walk along the hall to take the lift to the underground carpark was long, and I was finding it difficult to carry anything in my arms while trying to balance and walk at the same time. I was still seeing my neurologist once a year at St Vincent's Private Clinic in Sydney, and he had no real firm answers for me except to keep walking without aids. Over the period from 1991 to 2006 I had six MRIs, and had large doses of Botox injected into both my lower calf muscles to try and get more movement. There were no answers or treatment, but somehow both Greg and I continued to remain positive about our future.

I finally sold my Amaroo property in 2009, and I felt blessed as I had tripled the market price in the eleven years I had owned it. Greg and I were still living in his Carnaby apartment, and we decided to try and find a home to replace my Amaroo property, but we were looking for something that was on flat terrain. After a few months with no luck, we saw a beautiful block of land in a suburb that was set around nature reserves, ponds and parklands. We loved the location, and when we had a look at the floor plan the builder intended to put on this gorgeous piece of land, we were sold, and we started the long and painstaking process of building. It was in a new upmarket suburb called Forde, close to Amaroo, and this was appealing to us because we both were very fond of this area. We were excited, but dreading the building process and hoping everything would run smoothly.

We signed the contract on the 9th September 2009 and building commenced while we still lived in our Carnaby apartment. We were busy picking tiles, colours, kitchen and bathroom appliances etc. My mind was full all the time the building was taking place, and even though I would never build again, this was good for my relationship with Greg, because we were focused on a joint goal, and we were keen to live back on the ground, where the terrain was flat and we had an internal access garage, making life easier for my mobility issues.

We loved the floor plan, because we had grown-up children, and there was a room at the back of the house where they could get their privacy when they stayed overnight. Greg had his three children living away from Canberra, and I had Matthew living away, so this house was needed not only for us but to accommodate our grown-up children if they needed to stay.

We finally settled on our lovely new home in Forde on the 1st March 2010, and once it was finished I just burst into tears, as the stress had built up over the six months of the build and the many quick decisions I needed to make without much notice, and there was a lot of conflict with the builders. It got to a point where you just had to decide on what was worth fighting about and what was worth turning a blind eye to, because we were one of many who were building with this big company, and I found once the contract was signed, they didn't want to help or involve you much. The finished product worked out to be nice as I didn't like big homes. I found small homes more appealing for me, but the process was extremely stressful.

We were booked on another cruise in late February 2010, travelling with friends, and I couldn't wait to physically get away to try and reduce my stress levels and rest my mind from building our new home. On returning from our cruise we were able to move across from our Carnaby apartment with the help of a friend, and it was an easy move because I just picked up my clothes on their hangers and transferred them into the new wardrobe in our lovely new Forde home.

On the upside of our building and nearing the end, Chris and Linda were in full swing of building their first family home together in a suburb not far away from us and it was exciting to witness their build. It was very different from our experience as Chris was an owner builder and he and Linda had designed a beautiful, luxurious home with all the technical wizardry including a home theatre, music distribution throughout the house, a gorgeous spa/swimming pool and an alfresco outside area. Chris had started a building company with one of his best friends and they had decided on the name *Intrend*. They were building beautiful homes and on-selling them. The third company he set up was Comb Property Group Pty Ltd. They were using their gifts and talents they had developed since leaving college and completing their apprenticeships. As a family we were enjoying touring through their finished products. It was very impressive to see them achieving such a high standard of excellence and quality.

We decided to rent out our Carnaby apartment, and we had full intentions of keeping it as an investment property. It was in immaculate condition and we were hoping the tenants were looking after it, as we had wonderful memories of starting our married life in this lovely little home. It was sad in many ways to leave it.

My father's health had deteriorated, and he needed to come up to Canberra for a hospital admission to try and adjust his heart medication. He stayed in Canberra for a while after his discharge from hospital, and it was wonderful that my father had a chance to walk through our new home. He was very impressed with the building and floor plan. I was so proud of my father because he had been so healthy, fit and agile, but once he wasn't able to physically function he was accepting, and very interested in how our lives were going. I think he was in deep reflection of his own mortality and wanted to make sure I was happy and coping with life, especially after the loss of Richard, and my decline in health. He grew to really like Greg and was very impressed with his character and sincerity.

Once we were settled into our lovely new home and back on the ground, something was really missing for me. I had owned dogs all my life, and I started to look online for another Cavalier King Charles puppy, because I knew the temperament of this breed would be the best for me, as they are small dogs and easier to manage, especially with mobility issues. The next thing I had to do was convince Greg, because he had never had a dog and didn't feel the need for one. I found the most beautiful twelve-week-old Cavalier on-line and fell in love with his little face and superb markings. He was just perfect! He lived down in Berry NSW and I couldn't wait to get down to meet the breeders. I was hoping they would see that Greg and I would make good owners for this beautiful-looking little Cavalier. We finally met the one and only puppy the breeders were selling. They had intended to keep him because his markings were perfect and they wanted to show him, but as it turned out he wasn't going to be a tall or big Cavalier, and this was the reason they were now letting him go. We were able to assure the breeders that he would be living inside and this would be a forever home, so we were given the tick of approval. I was impressed with the way they screened us because it wasn't about money and they were not prepared to let him go unless he was going to a loving home.

In June 2010 we brought our beautiful puppy home to live with us, and we named him Jesse. He was already toilet trained and he enhanced our relationship because we could take him on walks together and he became such an important part of both our lives. We loved this little fellow so much, and as time went by I started to call him Bubba because he was so little, and Greg called him Louie, so in the end he answered to three names (Jesse-Bubba-Louie). He had the most amazing nature, and I found that with good eye contact I could discipline him well, so he was obedient. My walking was deteriorating gradually and I decided the only way I was going to enjoy the walks with Greg and Jesse was to invest in a mobility scooter. I decided on a little secondhand one, and it did the trick. It felt like magic to finally be able to enjoy going along with Greg and Jesse and to be able to look up and enjoy the scenery of our beautiful suburb and not have to look down to avoid a fall or a trip. I felt grateful, and to this day this red little mobility scooter has never let me down, as I am able to use it for distance where there is a lot of walking required.

On the 26th July 2010 we had the devastating news that my beloved father had passed away from heart failure. He lived down the south coast and it was good that both my sister and I, together with our sons, were able to visit my father the day before he passed. It was an emotional visit because my father was checking on us all. He went around, asking how we were all going and coping. It was as if he was saying his last farewells. His partner Betty wasn't making this emotional visit easy, by overriding the conversation, screaming and telling us that she had high blood pressure, and that our father was a selfish man because he didn't want to go into a nursing home. She was from Hong Kong, and we suspected she was only using our father for a home to live in. She had booked him into a nursing home, and he was due to move in the next day. I am convinced my father was broken-hearted, and I suspect he brought on a heart attack that night, preferring to die rather than having to live in a nursing home.

Betty met us at the hospital, and gave me a bag of clothes she wanted him dressed in, and things she wanted placed in his coffin (part of the Chinese culture). Both my sister and I were in total shock and hadn't even seen our father, and Betty was making all her demands on us. We were down the coast and had to take the opportunity to see the funeral director the same day to arrange my father's funeral, not to mention I had to drive back up the Clyde Mountain this same day after having hardly any sleep, in shock and grief. It was an enormous task for me emotionally. I never walked back into my father's home again, and none of the memorabilia that my father willed to my sister and me was ever given to us. He left his home for his partner Betty to live in for the rest of her life, bought her a car and left any money he had in the bank to her. I didn't care—as far as I was concerned she was out of our lives, and we didn't have to put up with all her lies and deception that she fed to my father the twelve years he was with her. I felt finally relieved to have her out of our lives.

We worked around the clock once we were back home, arranging my father's funeral, and my beloved father was buried at Batemans Bay just four days later. We were able to give him a beautiful celebration of his life on the 30th July 2010, and to this day I miss him beyond words. I often hear his voice and remember all the fun and laughter that he instilled in me as a child growing up. His instilling this into me in my formative years helped to make me who I am to this day. He had a charismatic personality, and was kind, and very engaging and affectionate to me as a little girl.

Greg and I returned home to try and enjoy our new little Jesse, and continued to love living in our brand new sun-drenched gorgeous Forde home. Krystal and Matthew were still living in Sydney, and often came home for the weekend, bringing their beloved Aussie. I found it distressing having the two dogs together, as Jesse was only a puppy and kept jumping up at Aussie. I wasn't able to cope, due to the trauma that I had with a bigger older dog mauling my chihuahua when I was fourteen, so to make this work we bought some fencing to keep Aussie and Jesse in separate areas.

Greg and I continued to do our cruising, and life was good to us both. We did a fabulous cruise to New Zealand, and later the same year we did a wonderful cruise called the Top End, departing from Sydney and docking in Brisbane, Cairns, Darwin, across to Bali, then back down to Port Headland, Geraldton, and ending in Fremantle. We enjoyed cruising with really good friends, and we were averaging two cruises a year, which was tremendous, living the life we had both envisaged. We were free spirits, and loved doing concerts, cruises and live productions on the spur of the moment.

In 2011, Chris and Linda were successful in establishing their third Wokitup store and extending their delicious creative menus to the south side of Canberra. It was another exciting and proud day for me as I watched this beautiful young couple work so hard to take risks to make their dreams happen. Wokitup Erindale was open for business on the 28th May 2011 with the full support of their families and friends. Another south side Wokitup followed in 2012 with Phillip Wokitup. It was exciting and wonderful to have my mother alive and in good health to see her grandson Chris complete his third and fourth Wokitup shops.

On the 7th January 2012, Matthew sent me a text from Sydney saying, "Suk guess what?" (Suk is his pet name for me.) I looked at this text and felt sick, hoping everything was all right. They were still trying to get the TallShip business up and running, and Krystal was supportive and was earning the constant wage. I couldn't answer his text for quite some time, but eventually sent him a text saying, "What?"

He came back with the exciting news that he had proposed to Krystal and she had accepted. I felt a tremendous relief! The proposal was very romantic, with a treasure hunt that Krystal had to go on all day long. He had signs leading to a park, and she was to find another note where there was some money to go and buy a new dress, that led to a romantic dinner, and then another sign saying, "fruits of your labour", and she had to dig in the garden, where there was one box inside another and another till she was to find his proposal. I felt very excited for them both, as I could see how much they loved each other, and Krystal was loyal and supportive of Matthew with this big change and risk they were taking with the TallShip venture.

We were able to go up to Sydney later in the January and arrange a surprise engagement dinner/party with a few friends who lived in Sydney. My sister and her husband travelled up, and my friends Lyn and John were delighted to come. Andrew, my sister's son, was living with Krystal and Matthew, so it was wonderful he was there. He is like a big brother to Matthew. One of Matthew's best friends, Ryan, and his wife, Erin, with their two little boys, Archie and Elijah, who lived in Canberra, were also at this wonderful celebration of Matthew and Krystal's engagement.

In the meantime, Aussie was rapidly declining in health, suffering with dementia, incontinence and blindness. Matthew and Krystal knew the end was near, and it was heartbreaking for them when it came time to say goodbye to Krystal's beloved Aussie, whom she had loved and cared for all his life. They flew up to Krystal's parents' home to spread his ashes and say their goodbyes. Anyone who has owned and loved animals would know they become a family member, and the grief of their loss is intense.

Matthew was finding quite a few of the other founding partners were not competent when he was working the long hours at TallShip, and he was becoming disillusioned. He decided to apply for a position in Department of Industry, Innovation and Science, and eventually received a response, with a subsequent interview via teleconference. He was successful in gaining this position, and so in May 2012 he moved back to Canberra to take up his new position. Krystal was able to join him, and our Carnaby apartment lease was ending, so the timing was good for them to move in and start a new chapter of their life together as an engaged couple. Krystal had come down to Canberra and set up their new abode, making it very homely and having their belongings around them. Krystal has a very nurturing and loyal nature and I felt Matthew was blessed to have a fiancée who loved, cared for, and supported him so much.

It was wonderful for Greg and me to have family living in Carnaby again (rather than tenants), as we had made it our first home after getting married in 2007. Krystal was also successful in gaining a permanent position in the Department of Health.

2012 was proving to be an exciting year for me as Matthew had returned to live in Canberra after four years away, with both him and Krystal securing permanent positions within the Public Service where they could maximise the benefits of their university degrees that they had both worked hard for.

As a mother all you want is to see your children doing what they love and are gifted to do and have a loving companion to enhance their lives. Everything I had ever dreamed of was now a reality with both Chris and Matthew taking risks and pursuing their dreams and working towards a future with the partners of their choice, complementing one another.

Matthew and Krystal had set their wedding date for the 26th October while they were busy working and living in Carnaby apartment and things were going well for all our family. I was still perplexed about my mobility and it seemed to be a slow downhill run with avoiding trips and falls and I still had no answers. I saw a small complex of ten independent villas on a plan proposed for a nice piece of land in the last stage of our lovely suburb of Forde. I took more interest in them because one unit was planned to be bigger for adaptable living with the wider hallway and doors. I also had a great interest in real estate and loved buying off the plan.

I was one of the first to see this proposed site and the artist's impression, and was excited about this boutique style of living. I felt I was replacing my gorgeous Amaroo property, and even better still, it would be on flat terrain. Subconsciously I think I was envisaging Greg's and my future, because I had no idea what was happening to my mobility and was concerned that maybe I would need the wider doors and hallways.

I said casually to Chris, "I think I am going to sell Carnaby," and to my surprise he said, "What do you want for it?"

I knew if I was going to put in an offer for the adaptable villa in this new upcoming lifestyle in Cassula Villas, I was going to need the funds to build off the plan. I was very keen because it was just a piece of land and I knew I would be able to offer below their asking price before construction had begun. With Chris now buying Carnaby I was able to put a bid in for twenty thousand dollars below the builder's asking price, and I felt confident they would accept this offer. To my delight my offer was accepted, and Greg and I were very excited to change our investment property from Carnaby to Cassula Villas.

This was another project Greg and I enjoyed together. We loved driving past each day and watching this gorgeous little boutique complex of ten villas coming together nicely. I was able to add a few extras, with more drawers and a bin cupboard in the kitchen, plus tiles put in the lovely wide hallway. It was a plan B in case Greg and I ever decided we needed to move in because we needed the wider doors and passageway, and flat terrain.

In March 2013, Wokitup number five, with another beautiful fit out, was open and ready for business in Braddon, to service the CBD of Canberra, and both my mother and sister were able to come and have a look before it was opened to the public. As much as I was excited for Chris and Linda, I was extremely relieved that they had decided to franchise and they were training up the new owners. I was missing Richard on so many levels as I felt responsible for encouraging, protecting and guiding Chris and Matthew through their beautiful young lives, and I missed not having him to share all these wonderful milestones that both our sons were achieving. I don't think I could ever explain the feelings I had; it was a mixture of excitement, pride and deep sadness that the children we had brought into this world didn't have both their parents to share their achievements. Having my mother was extremely important to me, because she also wanted the very best for Chris and Matthew. She was rock-solid in her support for everything they were doing, and was so involved, excited and interested! I knew she had my back and theirs in every aspect of our lives. I thanked God she was still healthy, sharp and very with it, because I really needed her more than ever.

Chapter 18
Joy and Sorrow

In late April 2013 I was delighted to have an unexpected visit from Matthew. He was looking refreshed and had a real glow to his face. We were both in my kitchen when he announced that Krystal and he were expecting a baby. It was a surreal feeling and it was as if he was four years old and telling me he was going to be a father! I couldn't process it, and was in some sort of disbelief and shock. It was such a strange feeling, that I couldn't put into words. All I could think of was that they had their wedding date set, and they needed to either bring the wedding forward, or relax and enjoy this pregnancy and have the wedding after the baby was born. I was so unprepared! If Matthew had told me beforehand that he was coming over to tell me something, I might have responded differently. Eventually it did sink in and I was beyond overjoyed, and for the first time realised I was going to be a grandmother, and had always wondered what that would be like.

My mother had always told me, "You wait till you become a grandmother!" I used to say to her I could never love a grandchild like my own children, and never really gave it much thought, but she would always insist that the love for your grandchildren is very protective and as deep a love as for your own children.

My mind was still reeling when Matthew left, and I was trying to process everything. This precious new life that Krystal and Matthew had created was very much planned, and they thought it might take some time, so they had decided they would start trying leading up to the wedding and conceive around their honeymoon.

All our family were very excited about having a new baby in our family, and Krystal's pregnancy was going along well. It was going to be wonderful for my mother as she was going to become a great-grandmother, and Mum and I would often talk about being grandmothers together. Krystal and Matthew had decided they were going to find out what sex their baby would be but keep the name they chose a surprise. The expected date was the 1st January 2014, and at twenty weeks they finally revealed they were expecting a precious little girl. I was excited to be having a granddaughter, especially as I didn't have a daughter, but most of all I prayed for their baby to be healthy and for Krystal's health to stay well and to have no complications.

The 20th of September 2013 was like any other day, but nothing could prepare me for the devastating news I was about to receive. Greg and I were going about our lives and I praise God we were in the A.C.T. We had just stopped to have a coffee break after doing some shopping when my phone rang. It was my sister's husband Laurie calling me to say that my mother had just had a stroke. He seemed calm and it didn't appear serious. I couldn't wait to get to the hospital and see how my mother was. My mother appeared quite good in her spirits when we arrived at Emergency, but I could hear that her speech was slurred. We were in Emergency and there were plenty of medical professionals coming in and out to assess my mother. It took hours to finally have her admitted into hospital, and it was a relief to know we would learn more about her condition and that she would be more comfortable.

I was devastated when I realised my mother was paralysed in her right arm, she couldn't speak clearly, and her cognition was impaired. She could only take in small amounts of information, and she was hooked up to a feeding tube. Her spirits were still very much alive, and she was laughing and very keen to get well and move into recovery. Her gold bangles were taken off her in the hospital and given to me. I brought them home and left them on my kitchen bench, hoping my mother would have a good recovery.

I started to feel anxiety as I had never before, because this was my mother whom I dearly loved and adored, and we had our beautiful little Jesse who was three years old, and I wondered how on earth were we going to be with my mother for long lengths of time and leave Jesse. He was an indoor puppy who didn't know life without having us around.

Then I thought of a lovely couple we had seen around in Forde while walking Jesse. They had a King Charles Cavalier dog previously, and I thought I knew where they lived in Forde. I sent Greg to their letterbox, hoping it was their home, to leave a note to say my mother had a stroke and was there any chance we could leave Jesse with them now and again until my mother was back home and recovered.

My mother stayed on the ward in the hospital until they could assess what damage the stroke had done to her. She was transferred to a rehabilitation ward and the slow journey of recovery began. My sister and I, with our husbands, were in to help my mother learn how to eat and dress herself, doing everything with her left hand, as the right arm was paralysed and she was unable to use it. Her speech was very slurred and she wasn't showing signs that she would be able to live back in her own apartment and be able to function. I was proud of my strong-willed mother who was working hard to recover, and I felt blessed she was still able to walk using a walker.

I was suffering severe heartache and shock, and found myself crying a lot. One morning I got up and saw my mother's bangles that had sat on my kitchen bench for weeks, and in deep grief and pain I picked them up and held them to my heart and just sobbed and sobbed uncontrollably. It was devastating and I was in a great deal of grief because I knew this was the start of all our lives changing, and I wasn't sure how my mother would cope with being dependent after being very independent, dominating, and always wanting things to be done her way. This was going to test us all as a family in very different ways.

A meeting was set up with my mother's specialists, and we were told we had to try and find a vacancy in a nursing home for my mother to live in. I had no idea of the hospital system or the aged care system, and we were really made to believe we had to look for a nursing home as soon as possible. My mother couldn't live with us, as I was struggling with unexplained mobility issues and hemifacial dystonia where I was coping with a constant spasm in the right side of my face, neck, throat, head and eye. I felt under tremendous pressure to find a nursing home that had a room for my mother. My sister and I had her enduring Power of Attorney but we were both inexperienced in the pressure the hospitals put on families to find a place for a loved one to live. We had to submit all my mother's details of her assets to Centrelink and it was expected we would have a rushed sale of my mother's home in order to secure a nursing home facility that would offer her a room. My sister and I went all over the A.C.T. placing applications into every nursing home.

We needed to clear out our mother's apartment and get it ready for sale, as the sooner we had the funds, the more chance we had of paying for a nursing home. My mother was a collector of fine china and jewellery, and had a room full of expensive collectors' items. I will never forget the day I had to ring up an auctioneer, and he came and opened all my mother's collector items over a full day. My mother was there watching on, but he knew we were very vulnerable and needed to try and get my mother's apartment up for sale. After a full day of him looking at everything, he offered $2,000 for the whole lot. He had young men waiting downstairs to take everything away quickly. I didn't have any idea how much any of my mother's collection was worth, but we all agreed we needed to let it all go, even though we knew he was going to re-sell everything and make a lot of money. My beautiful mother was so unwell—she was a shell of her old self—and it broke my heart to have to make such a drastic decision. My sister Maree and her husband Laurie as well as my husband Greg were there, and we all knew we had no other option.

We were finally offered a room in a nursing home, and we all worked hard to make this basic room feel like a home for my mother, with her belongings and furniture around her. It was not the ideal place, but we were all naïve and uneducated about the aged care system and how it works.

This was the beginning of a nightmare for my mother and all our family, as my mother was hysterical all the time. She was still able to use a phone to some degree, but often couldn't dial the correct number and couldn't comprehend a conversation due to cognition impairment. She screamed all the time, "Get me out of here!" My elder son found faeces under her toilet roll holder, and this was the start of finding a nicer, more modern, facility for my mother.

I found the aged care system to be complex and difficult to navigate and an ongoing cause of consternation. The so-called waiting list didn't exist. I found a small boutique nursing home that looked like a picture, and thought my mother would be safe, and happy to live there. I was told that there was no room for my mother, but interestingly, once I handed in the application and Centrelink assets details, I received a phone call, before I could even reach my home, that they had a room after all. It was then I realised that securing a room all depended on what a person's overall financial status was. I felt disgusted with the whole system but desperate to have my mother living in a much nicer facility, so I had to stoop to their level to agree. Again, we found ourselves moving all the beautiful furniture my mother owned, and making a homely place for her. I thought this was the beginning of keeping my mother safe, happy and well looked after.

Little did I know this was the start to another nightmare of distress, turmoil, and more devastation to come. We were all exhausted and I was receiving an onslaught of phone calls any time of the day or night from my distressed mother. I, my sister, and our husbands were visiting her, taking her out and doing everything and anything we could to help her cope and adjust to these new living arrangements. I was suffering from sheer exhaustion and stress from phone calls that made no sense, and I was jumping in the car at all hours of the day and night to get across to help and give comfort to my beloved mother.

In the early hours of the morning at 2.00 am on the 28th December 2013, I went to bed and for the first time turned our phones onto "Do not disturb" because I wasn't getting any sleep or coping.

Chapter 19

New Life and Twilight Years

At 10.00 am on the 28th December 2013, I felt ready to face the world again and turned on the telephones. To my great surprise, excitement, regret, and a whole mixture of emotions, I could see all the missed calls and messages from Matthew, that his and Krystal's precious and beautiful daughter had been born at 3.30 am. I felt devastated! I wasn't able to be at the hospital straight after her birth, as it never occurred to me when I turned the telephones off that my granddaughter would be born that very morning. My mind and body were exhausted from three-and-a-half months of hospital visits and rehabilitation, and then moving my mother into two successive nursing facilities, not to mention dealing with volumes of applications and contracts, and trying to get my mother's home cleared out and up for sale.

My sister and I were frantically trying to deal with Centrelink and endless paperwork, not to mention our mother's distressed and hysterical behaviour.

I was grateful Chris and his wife Linda had their phones on and were able to enjoy the excitement of Behati's grand arrival into our world. This gave me some consolation because I was distressed and disappointed that I wasn't there for Matthew at one of the most exciting times of his life. It was as if the whole world stopped on the

28th December 2013, and I couldn't wait to get to the hospital to see my first grandchild.

Matthew and Krystal were over the moon and I was delighted and excited to hold Behati for the first time. She was a picture of divine health and had a head of beautiful dark hair. I felt so emotional as I nursed her for the first time, and shed tears of pure joy, excitement and sheer relief that she was healthy and well.

Nursing Behati brought a flood of amazing memories, as she was born on the same day as Christopher. I loved having my son and now granddaughter share the same birthdate and couldn't help wondering if my faith in God had something to do with this, sending us a sign from Richard to let us know he was at peace! Krystal had a fast labour that was very intense and they only made it to the hospital by thirty minutes before Behati was delivered. I was relieved Krystal had her mother staying with them leading up to the birth, and knowing they had an experienced and loving mother with them was such an enormous blessing. This was the start of a beautiful new life, and it was exciting to see Krystal and Matthew bring home their beautiful daughter and see them become first time parents.

I was in emotional pain that Richard wasn't alive to see the birth of his first grandchild. I felt deeply for Matthew but I had to keep positive because all I wanted to see was them coping as new parents, and that the feeding and supply of milk went well. I also knew it was important that Behati was a settled baby because it makes the whole experience of parenthood amazing.

I also had to stay calm and keep things in perspective, because my mother was a handful and she had to make some big adjustments to living without her once great health. She needed much help and support. I was still grieving because my mother was no longer able to cope after having such an enormous stroke and bleed to her brain. The future looked bleak for her, and I was caught between grief and anticipation of my mother's passing away. It was difficult to describe how I was feeling, because I was overjoyed at the arrival of my first grandchild, but also sad from the loss of my mother's good health, and the thought of her ongoing care. My mother needed me more than ever now.

Greg and I were still following the building of our Cassula Villa when Matthew enquired about it. It wasn't a straightforward process, because we had taken it to exchange of contract, and Matthew and Krystal were going to take it to settlement. After a complicated legal process, they received the first home buyer's grant and stamp duty concession. They moved into their number 10 villa in February 2014 with their beautiful daughter Behati. It was exciting to see them buying their own first home, and Krystal made a gorgeous nursery, working hard to create a magical room painting, a feature wall and creative artwork.

Behati was blessed to have two parents to love and nurture her. I was overjoyed and excited to see them as a happy and contented family.

I couldn't have done more for my mother. I tried everything in an effort to settle her emotional state, always going to see her, but what had seemed like a beautiful nursing home soon turned out to be a nightmare. My mother's room was the farthest away from the nurses' station, and I was concerned when she was having falls, and it took a long time for anyone to find her. My mother was assessed by the aged care assessment team as high care, and this meant she needed more support and help. I was even more concerned when I realised my mother could take herself out of the facility whenever she wanted to go. I spoke to the manager, and I was told it was her right and they couldn't stop her from going for a walk away from the facility. I strongly disagreed because of her safety.

She decided to go for a walk one day at peak hour, and she had an enormous fall. She was a bruised and battered mess from the fall, having hit her body and face on concrete at the local shops. I felt at a loss about what to do. I found out that at night they had only one carer on duty to keep an eye on the residents. This was a disgrace, as there was no registered nurse on during the evenings.

My mother had a beautiful room and everything looked perfect, but I soon found out there was no care. My mother could talk in slurred speech and I was able to understand every word. I was horrified to find out they dragged her out of bed on some occasions to shower her at 4.00 am so they could get all the work done on skeleton staff levels. My mother was distressed, and she never stopped ringing me in a distressed state, needing me to help her. This was heartbreaking for me as well as for my beautiful mother. My sister and I agreed we had no choice but to get her out of this nursing home.

I had been advocating for eight months to get her into Goodwin Ainslie, and it was a battle talking to the admissions officer, developing an ongoing relationship with her so she knew we were keen as a family to have our mother in this facility. Securing a bed in this facility, which had a very good reputation, was like finding a needle in a haystack. This was my preferred nursing home, and I had delivered an application to them for a bed vacancy for my mother when she first had the stroke, but there was at least an eight-month wait.

Greg and I continued to try and do little things for ourselves during this trying time. We loved our little Jesse, and it was wonderful that the nursing home allowed us to bring him with us, so I felt relieved that he wasn't home alone. We developed a close relationship with the people who minded him and they could continue to have him when we couldn't take him with us, and that gave me peace of mind. We did little road trips away during this time and didn't stay away for long, but the breaks sustained us and gave us some respite from the ongoing care and attention my mother required. We were very relieved when we were able to get across to Mudgee and have a Christmas with Greg's daughters, their partners and his grandchildren.

Everything was a real balancing act between my time and energy levels. I was delighted that Krystal brought my beautiful little Behati around once a week on a Thursday so I could bond with her and spend quality time with her. I was relieved my health was holding up with the help from Greg. Having Behati was the only real, true joy I had in my life at this stage and it was delightful every time she came over. I just adored being a grandmother. Behati truly was a gift from God!

I received a phone call from Goodwin Homes that they finally had a bed for my mother. We took Mum to see Goodwin, and after she had another fall, my sister and I were relieved to be getting her into something safer, bigger and with more care. Unfortunately, my mother didn't cope and was screaming and lashing out at us to get her out. I realised nothing was going to make my mother happy, but there was a more senior carer who kept giving me hope by saying she would settle eventually. She was experienced with this type of reaction and behaviour.

It was traumatic to hear my mother swearing and abusing us no matter what we did. I couldn't switch off and I realised I was like that same little girl that used to always try and help both my mother and father when their behaviour was out of control in an alcoholic environment.

My sister was doing pastoral care at another aged care facility and even though it was new I had gone through it one weekend and had noticed there wasn't much care. I found a resident in distress. I couldn't find anyone to help this poor lady.

We had signed a contract with Goodwin Homes and we had decided we couldn't move our mother again. We were all exhausted and worn out. With my mother not settling after a week, my sister jumped at the chance when she received a call to say they could take her to the nursing home where she was doing pastoral care. I was beside myself, not believing another move was in the best interests of my mother.

I had a talk with my mother and pleaded with her not to move, but she believed, because she had seen a large bookshelf and a small sitting room outside her room, that this was her own library and sitting room. I felt sick because I knew the meals were brought up frozen from Wollongong and not cooked at the facility. I also was led to believe this was a new aged care facility run by people who had no experience in aged care nursing homes. The company was well known for over fifty-fives, and it had a good name for this type of living, but as far as a nursing home providing care to very vulnerable people, it was their first attempt within the A.C.T. I told my mother she was going from the frying pan into the fire and would be worse off. I also explained how difficult it was to get into Goodwin Homes. I had worked so hard over eight months to get my mother into the facility that I thought offered the best care, and had built up solid relationships with some of the staff with whom I was in regular contact. It felt as if it was all about to come crashing down and it did.

Chapter 20

Rollercoaster

I had worked so hard for so long to get a bed in Goodwin Ainslie, and there it was slipping away; we had just signed a contract and the management was not impressed. I felt I had nothing left, and collapsed into bed with depression and exhaustion for four days. I was angry and felt I was now going to have to settle my mother into yet another nursing facility. Her cognition was impaired, and all the abusive behaviour was the result of the stroke and her own frustrations. This decision to allow her to go to another nursing home had divided my sister and me in more ways than one. We had to find a way through—it was a rollercoaster ride we were on, and it was about to accelerate.

My mother had a lovely room and a balcony, and it had all the bells and whistles, but that was as far as it went. When you needed to speak to anyone you only had an answering service and no one returned your call. I couldn't get a carer to understand a basic word when asking for a toilet roll, so it was even harder for my mother with her slurred speech. So many carers were from a non-English-speaking country and it made communicating very difficult. My mother was still able to dress herself and she would be waiting for me with the words, "I am sitting here like a shag on a rock."

I used to take her for drives in the car to try and break up her day, but taking her back, knowing she was so lonely and unhappy, broke my heart. She ate the heated up frozen meals at the dining room with the other residents, and there wasn't a soul there that could be company or be a friend to her. It was a sterile and cold environment to say the least.

My mother continued with the same behaviour and aggression but this time it was more directed at my sister, because she was the one who had taken her there to look and moved her in. I had decided to step back from this move because I didn't believe it was in my mother's best interests, and knew it was an emotional ticking time bomb. My mother pleaded with me to get her back to Goodwin, but once you release a bed and have signed a contract, the management washes their hands of you and your family, and on this occasion I couldn't blame them. I did go to a meeting with Goodwin, but they made it very clear they didn't want to do business with our family, even though they could see clearly I was distressed. I was crying and apologetic because I had nothing to do with this decision to move her.

My mother continued to call me non-stop and it was difficult to understand her over the phone. My sister and I were doing everything we could but it was the same distressed behaviour. Due to the lack of staff, my mother was having some really bad falls. One carer had left her out on her balcony and forgotten about her, and my mother tried to come inside but had a terrible fall. She was left lying on the balcony for a very long time, and only by chance someone below on a walking path heard her calling out, and were able to go to the front office to alert them to my mother's dilemma.

I found this facility worse because they never called an ambulance on all the falls my mother was having. In fact, one fall warranted stitches, where she had fallen and cut her eyebrow, and I never knew about it. To this day my mother has a terrible scar above her eye. I could tell my mother didn't verbally attack me anymore and tried her best to behave when I was with her, because she knew that she and my sister had made this decision themselves.

I was struggling to get a car park close enough at this facility, and found it difficult because of my own impaired mobility. Greg was an enormous help and somehow we managed to find a way through. I was getting disturbed by the number of falls my mother was having, and at no stage did I receive a call from the nursing facility to alert me to them. I was finding out and seeing for myself the bloodstained carpet where my mother had fallen into the metal doorjamb.

She kept pleading with me, "Please don't let me die in this place!" and I reassured her I would try and get her out, but I knew I had exhausted every other option. I told her over and over again that if she didn't settle down, she was heading for another stroke, and I said to her there are worse things than death. She was swearing and cursing my sister and her husband for taking her there, and with the amount of emotional stress she was under, I could see clearly this was not going to end well.

I never received any calls from this nursing home, because my name wasn't even recorded on the contract papers. One night they rang my sister to say our mother had had another fall. I didn't know anything about it, and found out to my horror, but not to my surprise, that my mother was put to bed with a stroke, and they thought it was just another fall! Again, typical negligence, and lack of good and qualified staff to know the difference between a fall and a stroke, and that an ambulance should have been called.

I went straight to the hospital and found my beloved mother lying in a stroke unit. She had lost the ability to use her legs, and could only swing one arm, and that was to slap and/or lash out. The whole scene felt like a horror movie, with her aggression and ongoing swearing. She wasn't able to feed herself anymore, and we were all overwhelmed. Because she had a bed in a nursing facility, I knew it wouldn't be long and she would be transferred back to the nursing home.

I had to think quickly because there was no way she was going back into this nursing home in a worse condition—as far as I was concerned, they couldn't even look after her when she could walk, talk, dress and feed herself. I knew now I had to go back into action and take on the hospital system, because they want people to free up the beds, and I was dealing with a system that was brutal.

I said, "She is not going to ever return to the nursing home," and I took my story to ADACAS (A.C.T. Disability Aged and Carer Advocacy Service) in the hope they would delegate an advocate to help me keep my mother in hospital until I could find a nursing home that had capacity to deal with my mother's higher needs.

It was distressing for everyone, that because her cognition was now further impaired, she was now in nappies. She would look at me expressing she needed to go to the toilet but I would have to tell my mother she has to go in her nappy now. She needed lifting into a bed chair and into a bed. I asked my sister to release my mother's bed so the hospital didn't have the power to send her in an ambulance back to the same nursing home. I wasn't popular within the hospital system because I kept saying she couldn't go home because she doesn't have anywhere to go.

I was very stressed waiting for ADACAS to get back to me to see if our situation warranted an advocate to help me navigate the hospital system and their policies. To my delight and relief I received a call to say they took my story to an ADACAS weekly meeting and they gave us a really nice gentleman called Karl to help me endure meetings with my mother's medical team and social workers. The pressure to have my mother out of the hospital was an ongoing stress. I have never felt so determined in my whole life. I knew my rights and would not be backing down until I could find a nursing facility that would be able to cope and treat my mother with respect and dignity. I had seen so many nursing home facilities that don't allow the bed chair residents to be out among the other residents and I knew my mother wouldn't cope or last if she got stuck in a bedroom all day and night.

Just before Christmas December 2014, I was feeding my mother one night when two social workers came to see me. They applied pressure, saying my mother would be taken down to the South Coast and/or to Yass if I couldn't find a local nursing home. I felt angry but didn't show it and said, "Yes, she is going when I find the right aged care facility that can accept her new high care needs and has a vacancy." I knew what they were trying to do to me but I also knew I wouldn't crack when it came to a human rights issue and especially because it involved my mother!

I had the fight of my life battling the hospital system. My mother was still in hospital and my sister and our husbands and I were expected to be in a weekly meeting with the medical professionals and social workers to allow them to see we were a family trying to get a nursing home placement for our mother. Karl was an amazing advocate and support. He explained how my sister and I had to put on a united front at all times, so these specialists and the hierarchy of the hospital system couldn't see any cracks in our resolve.

When the hospital gave us a name of a vacancy at a nursing home we were expected to physically go and look at it, to prove to them we were serious about taking our mother out of the hospital system. I will never forget going to one nursing home which was a disgrace. It was very unclean and the people in bed chairs were placed in an unsafe area where people with dementia were allowed to roam around everywhere. I was quick to tell the hospital hierarchy I wouldn't leave my dog in there and I know they didn't like my decision that my mother would not be leaving.

Because we were away so much feeding our mother in the hospital our little Jesse had to be left with our good friends or he stayed home alone. You had to get into the hospital to feed your loved ones who couldn't help themselves because the meals were put in front of them and just left and there was no one to feed my mother.

I had an application in a nursing home that was a thirty-minute drive away from us on the south side of Canberra. I was impressed because they had a policy that everyone was to be out of their rooms every day including the people who had to live their lives in a bed chair. They also had a safe area for people with dementia so they couldn't attack or hurt a resident that was helpless or paralysed in a bed chair. My sister and I were very keen on this facility and we kept in regular contact with the administrations officer, letting her know we were under pressure and felt quite desperate. Unfortunately, you have to wait until someone dies before you get an offer of a bed, and it isn't a quick process. Once a room becomes vacant (and there is no repainting of the room etc), you are really at their mercy, and if you don't take the room, you miss out.

Chapter 21
Wedding Bells and Miracles

We were heading into 2015 and my mother was still in hospital and becoming more and more aggressive and frustrated. There was still no sign of an offer of a placement from a nursing home, and we were still attending regular meetings with the hierarchy of the hospital.

Karl from ADACAS was still going to every meeting with us and the pressure was horrendous. We were ringing on a regular basis in hope there was a vacancy in our preferred nursing facility. My sister and I and our husbands where doing everything we could to comfort and feed our mother daily, and we were still on an enormous rollercoaster ride of emotions. It didn't look like ending any time soon.

Matthew and Krystal had set their wedding date for the 7th March 2015 and the excitement of this joyous occasion was keeping my spirits and hope alive. Krystal showed me the beautiful colour her bridesmaids would be wearing, and they were inviting some of my friends. That meant so much to me. I was getting very excited and feeling secure that I would be surrounded by some faithful and trusted friends on such a special day.

Behati was fifteen months old by this stage and she hardly slept so it was going to be a challenge to get her to have a sleep on this big and exciting day. Behati had a gorgeous dress to wear on such a special occasion. It was made to coordinate with the bridesmaids' colours. Everything was booked and it would be a beautiful garden wedding followed by an indoor reception that flowed out to a large alfresco area.

I was busy trying to get my outfit together, and wanted to do my son proud on his wedding day. I found a lovely Italian lace dress, and knew I could only cope with flat platinum sandals. I was concerned about my mobility, and found a slimline walking stick on-line to match my dress, and had it sent over from America. To my delight, it was a perfect colour match, with a small chrome handle. I felt it would look like an accessory from the Victorian era. I had found a makeup specialist near our home to make me look as good as possible. To be the mother of the groom was a privilege and an exciting time, and a day that I could look back on and be happy and proud.

I was hoping my mother would be offered a permanent place before the wedding so I could relax, but we were well and truly heading into late February and there was still no sign of a placement. I felt desperate because my mother's health was so poor I even thought we might be dealing with a marriage and a funeral at the same time.

I remember saying to my sister that if something was to happen to our mother we were just going to have to delay the funeral. I had got to the stage of being pragmatic about the whole situation.

I was working on my speech and thought this would be easier because more time had gone by since Richard had passed away. I was wrong. A flood of emotions kept making me feel sad for Matthew, and I wasn't as good with my mobility as I'd been when Chris had got married. I wondered how on earth was I going to deliver a speech on behalf of Richard and myself. I thought, here we go—another major milestone with Matthew getting married and a beautiful new daughter-in-law and granddaughter and I was hoping and believing Richard was there with us all in spirit. I felt deeply sad for Richard's father who was still alive but in failing health and I was pleased he was able to make it to the wedding ceremony. He wasn't well enough to stay for the reception.

I received a call from Matthew leading up to the wedding asking Greg and me to take Krystal to an after-hours doctor so he could stay home with Behati. I was concerned because Krystal had lost quite a bit of weight and I was hoping she would be well on the wedding day. She was diagnosed with a urinary tract infection and it was a relief to know that with the right medication she would be out of pain and able to recover in time for her wedding day. It was wonderful that Krystal had her mother and father in Canberra leading up to this special day because they all worked hard to make this a magical day by pulling all the fine details together.

Matthew and a friend arrived at our place one night to see if his dress suit still fitted him. He was really buzzing and it was delightful to witness because I knew Matthew, who was now thirty-two, was ready to take on the responsibility of being a husband. It was heart-warming to see both my sons finding true happiness and love especially after those tough and traumatic years. They had both done me proud to have kept strong and were making excellent decisions for their own lives. I had prayed and worked so hard to be there for them in any way I could so they could see and experience that life was to be cherished and embraced.

They had both grown into men of good character and depth with humility and empathy, and these important traits would take them through life and hold them in good stead for the future.

I wanted my mother, who had played a big part in all our lives, to be present to witness her youngest grandson making his wedding vows, but she was in such a bad place emotionally that I couldn't have a conversation with her. She was lashing out and the behaviour wasn't all to do with the stroke. I knew she would have enjoyed it as much as Chris's wedding. She loved her three grandsons so much and even though she came across as bossy and opinionated, she was very much interested to know all about their lives.

The 7th March 2015 arrived and we were all ready with great excitement and anticipation. Krystal looked stunning as her father walked her down the garden path to Matthew. The day was just perfect with no wind and beautiful sunshine. All the family members and friends witnessed this beautiful celebration of two lives coming together. I enjoyed listening to the celebrant and hearing what Matthew had written about what attracted him to his bride: Loyalty, Nurturing and Prettiness. It made it very intimate and personal. I knew my son well because he was deep and would be wanting these qualities in a life partner. He had won the jackpot because Krystal had them all and I knew she would always be faithful, honest and true to him.

Richard's sisters and their families were all present to witness this beautiful celebration. More time had passed since we had all lost Richard and there was more healing from our grief and pain. There is nothing like a marriage or a birth to bring everyone together in love and unity. It was a fabulous wedding and made even more special to see Matthew with his brother Christopher as best man and his cousin Andrew as his groomsman.

We didn't know we were about to get the biggest surprise and shock of our lives!

There was a silent miracle at their wedding, and just a few weeks after they were married, we were all elated to receive the news that a precious new life was growing, and Krystal and Matthew were going to become parents again. The due date was 18th November 2015! All was going well and the miracle of another new life was exciting. I was going to be a grandmother for the second time and I felt blessed. I had lost so much, and now the good Lord had given me two beautiful daughters-in-law, a gorgeous granddaughter, and another grandchild was on the way. Both Chris and Matthew had found their life partners, and I was given the most patient, caring and loving godly husband in Greg. How could I complain about anything?

I kept hearing God's promise, "And we know that in all things God works for the good of those who love him, who have been called according to His Purpose." (Romans 8:28).

Four days after the wedding, I knew without a doubt this was a real answer to prayer when we were finally offered a room in the nursing home we had been waiting on for my mother. At long last we could finally say goodbye to the hospital system and all the red tape and bullying tactics. We had waited over three months for this nursing home that we thought could offer a high level of care that my mother needed so badly.

My mother was transferred to the new nursing home, and I will never forget what she said: "I am only here for the day!"

I didn't argue, because I was just thanking God for finally giving me the one and only place that I thought could offer my mother the best care for her current state of health.

Chapter 22
Kids and Old Folk

The new nursing home had a homely feel and it was as though everyone lived in little cottages. I loved that all the meals were homemade in a kitchen on the premises and family members were encouraged to stay and have a meal with their loved ones. It wasn't a modern facility, but I was impressed that mostly everyone could speak English and there wasn't a big turnover of staff. Some staff had been working there for up to ten to twenty years, so there was stability.

My sister and I were so worn out we made a decision to leave the existing furniture they provided and to allow the facility to do all our mother's washing because we both had farther to travel to get to the nursing home on the southside of Canberra. We made our mother's room personal by putting up her own pictures and wall clock, lamps etc. My mother's cognition wasn't good, so she didn't notice the walls that needed painting and the stained carpet. That was a relief because she was a real perfectionist and would never approve if she could take it all in.

The aggressive behaviour was still there, and she was still going to fight this as long as she could because she just couldn't accept this was her new life. It was a relief that there were concerts, activities and church services to attend. She used to love shopping in this part of Canberra so it was good I could always tell her she was living close to her favourite shops. I was very impressed that there was a resident dog, an aquarium, birds and chooks outside. My mother enjoyed us wheeling her all around the facility, and she could watch and see plenty of activity. I needed Greg to help me because the bed chairs were very heavy and difficult to wheel. Jesse loved coming to every visit and was allowed off his lead and he ran everywhere. Jesse's lifestyle finally took a turn for the better; he was free at last! We had many requests for Jesse to do private room visits to residents that were bedbound, and Jesse uplifted their spirits by his ongoing visits, sitting on their beds while they could give him lots of cuddles. It was heart-warming.

My mother of course wasn't impressed because she wasn't an animal lover so at this stage he wasn't allowed on her lap.

We were able to have our own private room when we wanted to hold a private function for my mother, and she was delighted when the family were all together, especially to see her grandchildren Andrew, Chris and Matthew. She seemed to be the happiest when they were around her, but she didn't behave herself around my sister and me. My sister and I would often say our mother had more time for her grandchildren and we were both doing all the work. She was receiving a few visits from some of her friends and extended family members, so this was a time that really lit up her life.

Everything was going well for Krystal's health during her pregnancy and we were all looking forward to having another precious new life in our family. Krystal had returned to the workforce and was working three days a week. Behati was in childcare three days a week and was really struggling to adjust. I would have done anything to be safe and well enough on my feet to mind her instead of her going to childcare. I found I was having a lot of grief around becoming a grandmother because I wasn't well enough to mind Behati on my own, but I did all I could do to be grateful and try and stay positive. This was another time I relied heavily on my faith that Behati would be protected and cared for by the childcare workers.

Her childcare was in the same building Matthew worked in, so that gave me some peace of mind.

I was meeting up with my cousin every couple of weeks and he was diagnosed with a rare disease. We enjoyed our time together as his mother was my mother's sister and his father was my father's brother, making us double cousins. He was ten years younger than me but because we both were not working it was a chance to have quality time together. It was good for us both because I was a member of a closed Australian Dystonia Support Group and between my faith in God and the fact I had a support group I was coping as best I could.

I didn't quite understand what my cousin was suffering from but could relate because we were both struggling. I had so much faith, trust and respect in my specialist in Sydney whom I had seen since 1992, that I never questioned his diagnosis.

Life was tiring with the travel to and from the nursing home, and the time I spent with my mother didn't allow much time in my week, except to catch up with my cousin, or have a quick coffee and chat with a friend. I loved having Behati whenever I could. She was growing up so fast and she was adorable, with all this glorious thick curly hair, and she loved her time with Greg and me. I would often have a close friend come over the day Behati came to give us extra physical support. I loved playing with her as she had a vivid imagination and was such a strong-willed little girl. I could tell from an early age that she loved dolls and our dog Jesse and loved mothering them. She was very determined and was difficult to get to sleep. We would take her to feed the ducks, and afterwards Greg and I found ourselves walking for long periods to try and get her to sleep. I used to ride my scooter and Jesse was always with us. I was relieved that my health was holding up, and with the help of Greg and a close friend we managed somehow. Having Behati was what gave my life joy and purpose, because it was very difficult emotionally dealing with my mother's ongoing attacks of anger and verbal abuse. I could tell this behaviour was not going to go overnight but at least she was safe, clean and cared for.

2015 was turning out to be a much better year! We had found a church fellowship to belong to, and Greg was able to play music, which was and always will be his passion and his God-given talent. I was much more settled knowing my mother had a placement in our preferred nursing facility. Even though we still needed to be in the aged care facility to help her, at this stage she was still able to eat solid meals and the carers were able to feed her and give her fluids.

I was trying to come to terms with the fact that Chris and Linda might never become parents. I knew they had started IVF. I had severe heartache and pain. I admired them both because even though everyone was having babies around them, they always remained so excited and happy for all their friends, and Chris was very excited for his brother. Here they were; so successful in business and had made some wise decisions that put them on their feet financially, and yet it looked as if they would probably never have a child of their own.

Matthew asked Greg and me if we would like to go with him and Krystal for the twenty week scan as they had decided to find out the sex of their baby but leave the name for a surprise for everyone. We both felt honoured and delighted to be asked. Krystal and Matthew found out first and then we were invited in to see the scan. I couldn't tell whether they were having a boy or a girl but we were delighted to learn they were having a precious little boy. Greg and I had prayed this little miracle was healthy and indeed the scan showed everything was normal for Krystal and their son.

As we were drawing closer to November, it was good to know Krystal had her mother with her in the days leading up to the due date. I was concerned as they only made it to the hospital in the nick of time with Behati's birth, and I was hoping they would have more time before this delivery. I had my phones on day and night this time because I didn't want a repeat episode of not knowing about the birth till many hours later. There was going to be less than a two year gap between Behati and her little brother. I was praying they had a good birth and the baby would be feeding and sleeping well.

On November the 18th 2015 a beautiful baby boy arrived into our world and Matthew rang me to say Leo was born. Matthew's voice over the telephone was elated and he was telling us to come straight away. I was over the moon and couldn't wait to get to the hospital.

We drove as fast as we could but we were caught up in the early morning traffic. It was the best experience, because it was straight after the birth and Leo was just perfect in every way. He had fair hair and was with Krystal in the birthing suite. She had it booked till 5.30 pm that same day. Things were very different from when I had my boys and we stayed in hospital for at least a week, but I knew Krystal was capable and her father was arriving that same day so we enjoyed a little nurse with Leo. We didn't stay very long because Krystal's mother arrived with Behati. She was still young and needed to be with her parents and adjust to the idea that there was a precious new little brother in her life and world. It was a relief to see them all together and I know Matthew was really excited to have us there this time.

Greg and I hosted Christmas that same year in December 2015 and it was a blessing to have both my grandchildren at our home. I was delighted to have Richard's father come to our home for Christmas with his grandsons and great-grandchildren. He kept saying he hadn't long to live and I knew he was telling me the truth because he was unable to eat or drink much. He had struggled for decades after having a stomach operation due to ulcers caused by too much alcohol consumption.

There were twelve of us in total and because my health wasn't good, Greg and I had to work over a long period of time to decorate our home. Everyone contributed with the food preparation so that made it easier. I was still missing my mother more than anyone realised and I remember driving across to the nursing home on Christmas Eve just to be with her. There was a lovely church service on and it was special to go with her to that. I couldn't bring her home for Christmas Day because I couldn't fit a bed chair through my internal doors. Besides, when my mother could not comprehend what was happening around her, she would go off her head. I couldn't risk that behaviour and it would have disrupted the whole day, not to mention upsetting Behati who wasn't quite two years old at this stage

We were all moving into 2016 very well and there was great excitement when Chris and Linda opened up their sixth Wokitup shop in Amaroo and were training up the new franchisees. This was a lovely young couple who were enthusiastic, energetic and excited to be the owners of their own business. Chris had done a fabulous job in building them a beautiful shop. Linda was committed to staying with them for as long as it took to have them feeling confident and capable at running their own business.

Greg and I went for our seventh cruise, and we were relaxed and happy to have had a chance to get away on our own and have some much needed rest and relaxation. I kept in contact with my sister to make sure my mother was stable the whole time and we weren't far away if we needed to come home quickly. It was such a relief to know everything at the home front was calm and stable.

Chapter 23

Scars into Stars

We returned home feeling refreshed by our cruise and decided cruising was the best form of travel for us. Greg had spent years in Foreign Affairs travelling the world with his work and I felt I had seen enough of the world and because my mobility wasn't good we didn't want to put ourselves in a non-English speaking country. I adored Behati and Leo and they were both growing fast. It was such a relief that Leo had a very chilled out easy-going nature, making it a bit easier on both Krystal and Matthew because Behati was a strong-willed little girl. They were doing a great job finding a balance with their work and home life.

My mother was still struggling in care and my sister and I with our fantastic husbands were doing all we could to help her through each day. Sadly, some of her oldest friends who had come to visit her over a period of time became unwell themselves. I had the difficult task of having to tell my mother that certain friends had passed away, and I could tell she was shocked and upset by this. Life was fragile and I was trying to seize the moments with my mother.

In August 2016 Linda and Chris announced that they were expecting a baby and everyone was excited and thrilled for them. They had dated for eleven years before they were married and now they had been married twelve years and were expecting a baby via IVF. I was excited but also quite anxious the whole way through the pregnancy as I knew the risks with IVF babies. I had never in my whole life prayed so much for this wonderful couple to have their own baby. Linda was amazing, texting me and answering my texts, because this baby meant so much to me to finally see my elder son become a father. It was a real miracle as far as I was concerned and I believed God would bring forth this baby for them.

Linda was very confident from the start that all would go well. They decided they didn't want to know the sex because they said there weren't enough surprises in this world anymore. I know that as sick as my mother was, she was relieved to know that Chris would soon be a father. She was delighted to know that Matthew and Krystal were married and had a daughter and a son. I encouraged her so much to be grateful that she was seeing her grandsons grown up as husbands and now fathers, but I knew she was a proud and determined person and would have wanted to be able to enjoy her great-grandchildren while she was in good health. There was often a lot of tears of grief over this but she always pulled herself together to be the best she could be when they came in to visit her.

I had been receiving calls from the Canberra Hospital Genetics department because they were interested in taking a blood test to see if I had the same disease as my cousin. My sister had gone for genetic testing and her results had come back positive. I didn't take any of this seriously and neither did Greg, in fact we were both quite blasé. I had seen a neurologist from 1992 and it was now 2016. I had all the confidence, trust and respect in my treating neurologist and was an active member in a Dystonia Australian Support Group, and everything I was enduring in my body made sense when I read my specialist's reports and shared in my support group. Because Chris and Linda were doing IVF I started to think surely a blood test wouldn't hurt so I decided to visit a genetic clinic. I also thought I owed this to my children and grandchildren. My parents, grandparents and all the extended family that I knew of were all healthy and well, so both Greg and I were 100% sure that I didn't have a genetic disease.

Chris came along to listen to the genetic specialist. It was a short and simple appointment and I had the blood test and didn't think another thing about it. I was on my own when a call came through over four months later from a genetic counsellor to tell me I had Hereditary Spastic Paraplegia type 7. This had been genetically proved by the laboratory in Western Australia. SPG 7 is just one of the many conditions they test for. Both my parents carried the same two mutations within this gene. This condition is inherited in an autosomal recessive manner. This would make my children carriers but unless they are married to a carrier of a mutation in the same gene they could not have an affected child. The genetic clinic was offering to test Chris and Matthew's wives once they had my results.

I felt numb and couldn't talk to Greg or anybody for a few hours because I was trying to process this. What did it mean for my children and grandchildren? I felt sheer relief because it wasn't dominant and so I couldn't pass it on to them. I couldn't believe what I was hearing. I had struggled so hard to be believed by almost everyone in my life including my husband of twenty-nine years. They'd believed all the medical professionals who said my symptoms were psychosomatic, and had proceeded to gossip and put down my good reputation. I was a hard worker, honest and loyal and yet my whole life had fallen apart. I had lost my family home, my marriage, and the ability to live with my children because of Richard's decisions and beliefs about my condition. My conversion to Christianity and the intense work I was doing with my 12-step Al-Anon had saved me and I had a very resilient and determined nature.

I was referred to a HSP clinic at Royal North Shore Clinic where it was explained to me in more detail. I did have Dystonia, and they couldn't rule out that the violent reaction I had from the doses of Haloperidol might have interfered with the autonomic nervous system. The HSP was lying dormant in my body since I was born, but the interference had happened and this is when I started to notice a gradual decline in walking, causing tripping and falls.

My treating neurologist was relieved and supportive to hear of the new diagnosis and I still continued to see him because over the decades I had really grown to respect him. He was the only specialist who believed me and never wrote a negative report. He was right that I did have dystonia and it in itself was very difficult to cope and live with on a daily basis without also finding out I also had a rare genetic progressive disease.

I couldn't help wondering if Richard had understood or was told I had a progressive genetic disease, would he still be alive and with me. If that had happened, maybe things could have turned out differently. Still, my faith in God was so great that I knew God was in control of every aspect of my life and he was carrying me through all the tragedy, trauma and loss. God had brought Greg into my life to love and care for me unconditionally.

Both Greg and I were shocked and decided we were not going to allow this news to change the love and care we had for each other. We understood it was a progressive disease and that our lives were going to change in some enormous ways and we would have to find a way through it, doing things differently.

I decided to create a closed Facebook support group for people living within Australia who were suffering from HSP, to stop the isolation, disbelief and loneliness. I felt very passionate that no one needs to suffer in silence. I called it Hereditary Spastic Paraplegia Australian Support Group. I was very keen to run face to face gatherings of people who were suffering with the challenges of living with HSP to share quality time together in the different locations in Australia. I wanted to make a difference and help people through as best I could, because of the lack of help and difficult diagnosis. I wanted to bring awareness and understanding to such a rare and debilitating progressing disease. A support group was badly needed, especially within Australia.

I decided to contact an international HSP support group and put a post up asking if there are any Australians with HSP in one of these big international groups. I received a response from a few Australians and I looked at how big the groups were and felt we needed a HSP closed group for Australians only, so there was more chance of meeting each other face to face to talk about our feelings and the challenge it is to live with a rare genetic disease. This started with just me and one other Australian who was, like me, excited to find someone in the same situation. It was small beginnings and my primary purpose was to create a safe, secure and friendly group. I didn't understand HSP very well and as time went by I couldn't find many specialists who even knew about it.

It wasn't long before more people living with this disease were requesting to join at a slow and steady rate. We had admins to run and take care of the members' questions and we gained trust and respect in this friendly and warm little forum. It was so much nicer than the big international groups because we could share so many details about our symptoms, information and entitlements that the government were providing, specialists that knew about HSP and a whole array of related topics. Greg and I were able to do quite a few gatherings in different parts of Australia which were both confronting and rewarding, meeting so many amazing people who were inspirational, humble, and in spite of their difficult challenges were willing to share their lives with us.

Chapter 24
Faith, Hope and Joy

2017 was starting off to be a year of Celebration, Excitement and Success. I was turning sixty on the 29th January and I had decided I didn't want a big party. I was extremely tired from the ongoing care of my mother and the progression of HSP so we decided to have a celebration birthday party at our home with only immediate family. I was excited to have my dearly loved family around me, and I had a beautiful array of balloons delivered to give that celebration feel to my birthday party. I was loved and spoiled by Chris, Linda, Matthew and Krystal together with my gorgeous grandchildren Behati and Leo.

Maree and Laurie were keen and excited to celebrate such a milestone, especially after so much loss and trauma. Amazing how you really appreciate everyone who is in your life when you reach sixty and the journey to this age wasn't smooth sailing. I was very grateful that my immediate family understood that I just wanted something quiet on my actual birthday and then Greg and I were heading off for a week on Hamilton Island. We had booked romantic accommodation where it was expensive, but it was nice to be able to spoil ourselves with chauffeur-driven vehicles whenever we wanted to go and be picked up.

Greg and I couldn't believe how beautiful Hamilton Island was and we loved the fact we didn't have to leave our own country to feel such peace and relaxation.

I was keen to do the very first HSP support gathering in Brisbane, so we stopped over in Brisbane on our way up to Hamilton Island. It was exciting to meet some of our members from our new Australian HSP support group in person. A large number of people had HSP and it was amazing how we all felt so comfortable and relaxed with each other right from the beginning of our night together. We were able to compare and share many facets of our lives together and the limitations and challenges we were all facing, and yet everyone was positive and excited to be in each other's company. I felt respected and cared for because they had a large birthday cake all organised so I could celebrate my sixtieth birthday with them.

It was amazing; our Australian Support Group had not long started and here we were in Brisbane enjoying each other's company. My vision of how a support group should come to life was now a reality!

After we arrived back from Hamilton Island we had only a few months to wait until my third grandchild would be born. Linda was well and truly showing and she was happy and healthy through the whole pregnancy. It was exciting because there wasn't going to be much age gap between this little one and Leo. All I could think of was that Behati and Leo would have a precious cousin soon, and Chris and Linda would finally be parents. I couldn't believe it, that both my sons had made it through such trauma, the loss of their loving father and my health decline, and were both amazing husbands to their wives, and sons to me. I was elated that we were all still moving forward in our lives in a positive and productive way. They respected and loved Greg and could see he was such a wonderful husband to me and they knew he genuinely cared for their lives, happiness and wellbeing.

On 28th May, Linda gave birth to Chelsea by a rushed Caesarean section after a long and complicated labour, but the only thing that mattered was that both Linda and Chelsea were doing well. I was overwhelmed with excitement, and to see Chris for the first time after the birth was emotional, because he was so excited to have a beautiful healthy baby daughter. I could see he had been crying tears of sheer relief, excitement and joy. I couldn't begin to express the relief I felt that Chris and Linda were now parents. I'd had private deep grief that they may never experience parenthood, so this truly was a miracle and I was praising God because He was faithful to all my prayers and desires for both my sons and their families. Linda was able to feed beautiful little Chelsea without any complications and she was an easy baby, sleeping and feeding well.

My mother was relieved to know that Chris was a father and was going nowhere until she was well and truly ready. She had seen Matthew become a father twice and now Chris. It was something that she could only really share with me because she wasn't able to talk at this stage and I had a relationship with her that was becoming more and more beautiful. We had become closer emotionally and I understood everything she was expressing through her body language, nods, eye rolls and tears. We had a relationship that was raw, vulnerable, honest and transparent; something I had wanted from my mother all my life. All the barriers were gone and we were able to communicate and say things to each other that I'd never thought were possible. Caring for my mother at the end of life was an enormous privilege and there was so much beauty in our relationship, and even though others didn't comprehend it I knew this was another miracle from God. He knew my heart and knew my attachment to my mother and He was looking after my emotional wellbeing. My mother and I needed this time. My mother was now in acceptance, and even though the journey was heartbreaking and horrendous, she was finally making her peace with herself, God, and me. My mother had rebelled against the God of the Bible, and had gone into new age philosophies and seeking clairvoyants for tarot card readings. I had prayed for the salvation of her soul, and asked God to leave her on this earth until she was back with the one and only true God, who could offer eternal life. I had prayed my little heart out for my mother to end well, and despite what the world saw as success, I knew now that there was a hell and a heaven, and both my mother and I had spent years discussing this.

I was the last person she expected to hear talking about my faith, because I had been agnostic before my conversion to the Christian faith. I always said to her with tears flowing down my face, "I want you to be there on the other side when it is my turn."

I knew my father and Richard had made it, and I was going to be united with them. I wanted more than anything on this Earth that my mother, who I had always loved and adored so much, would be there too. I couldn't see the point of living this life and gaining all the fame, wealth and success, if your soul wasn't saved. I was once so dead to the spiritual realm, that I couldn't believe that out of suffering, the God of the Bible had rescued me, and I wanted to see all my family still living on the other side of death.

My mother and I had discussed in a way that she could comprehend with limited cognition that this world we were living in had abandoned God and gone their own ways without a moral compass. I spent these necessary and critical years since she had the strokes, sharing with her my relationship that I now had with a living and real God and she was beginning to realise how crucial it was that she didn't have an abrupt end to her life before she had a chance to call on the name of Jesus! I was finally seeing the seeds I had continued to sow into my mother's heart bearing fruit. Her heart was softening and she truly believed she would be reunited with all her loved ones that had died in Christ. I felt all the hours, days, months and years I was investing into my beloved mother's life were worth every minute. Not only was I feeding her physically but more importantly I was uplifting her spiritually and her own faith was increasing. It was exciting because I would play her Christian music and she would mouth the lyrics of the chorus. She was fading away physically before my eyes but growing in the spiritual realm and that was of the utmost importance to her and to me.

Susan Nicholson

Chapter 25

Success and Acceptance

Chris and Linda were still busy building their successful chain of franchised Wokitup eateries, and expanded into Queanbeyan NSW, my birthplace, in October 2017. Chelsea was only six months old and it was a pleasure to go with Chris and Chelsea to the grand opening day. Linda was already there because her role was to work with the new owners until they were confident and adjusted into running their own business. Once again Chris had built a grand shop and I was always interested in the fine detail of the fit out of all their shops.

Kippax Holt followed in December 2018 and it was in another part of Canberra where they would have regular customers and a continuous flow of clientele. Linda and Chris had the full support of their families and we were all excited for them.

I felt relieved because they now had Chelsea, and I didn't want to see them working so hard. I knew they would want to invest their time and energy into their beautiful daughter for whom they had waited so long. Chris was still building homes through his building company Intrend, and then keeping them in Comb Property Group. He had them in the rental market, so he had set himself and Linda up so that this was a separate company and had nothing to do with his Wokitup Franchised Eateries. They had kept one of their Wokitup shops as a Flagship for themselves, as they had to make all the variety of sauces from one kitchen to attain the same consistency and service the other franchised eateries. They were busy trialling new and innovative combinations of delicious foods and flavours, and bringing them into the other franchised shops.

Matthew founded Beleo Capital in 2018 to invest for friends and family across global markets, reducing portfolio risk as the world enters the last stages of a long term debt cycle. I was proud to see Matthew following his passions and what he was gifted and talented to do.

Greg and I minded Behati when we could, especially helping out in the school holidays, and we enjoyed taking her to movies and outings that were suitable for her age group. I loved setting up and doing craft activities with her, and she was growing up so fast and was happy spending time on her own with us. She enjoyed listening to stories about my childhood. She was deep, and emotionally very intelligent. I loved her so much and it was getting exciting because we were able to attend grandparent activities at her school. She was only five, but quietly confident, and she loved going to her school canteen with a little bit of her own money and buying what she wanted. Leo was occasionally coming around by himself at this stage of our lives. He was more reserved in his nature and was a very kind and caring little grandson. He was gifted and talented with sports and his fine motor skills were excellent and advanced for his age. He wanted to always share and include his big sister Behati. He liked to take something home to her when he was with us. Chelsea was now two, and we hadn't had her come and have any play dates by herself. However, she was coming with Chris and we really enjoyed her. I wasn't confident on my legs and knew I would have time once she was out of nappies and when I didn't have to lift her up. I struggled with the fact that back in 2013 when Behati was born I was stronger and able to walk without aids. I hoped my grandchildren would remember that I loved and cared for them, and would be able to overlook my limitations once they were older. Chelsea was advanced in her speech and she was confident and secure. She loved dancing and dressing up. I told Linda I thought Chelsea was made for the stage.

It was exciting to see their little God-given personalities developing, and I felt that Chris and Linda and Matthew and Krystal were in tune with my grandchildren's very different emotional needs. I loved being a grandmother, but was struggling emotionally with my diagnosis of HSP and the progression of this genetic disease. I kept telling myself I had to be grateful that I was able to raise my own children as best I could, and that I could enjoy my grandchildren, but I was still dealing with deep loss and grief, and was looking forward to seeking a grief counsellor. I was so time poor I couldn't see myself fitting in any more appointments while ever I was caring for my beloved mother. My mother was really struggling by this stage and even though she was slowly fading away she was determined to fight this and wasn't ready to say goodbye.

I was strongly advised by my physiotherapist that I was now a high falls risk, and that I had drop foot and had to be on a walker at all times. A scooter was required for longer distances.

I was on the NDIS (National Disability Insurance Scheme) by this time. It was proving to be beneficial, but quite daunting, because of the complexities of the system. It kept me busy, with hydrotherapy and gym work with an exercise physiologist, and I came home feeling fatigued. I wondered why, if there was no cure, I was putting myself through all this. It wasn't as though I was working on a knee or hip replacement. I also knew that the only thing that might keep the progression of this disease at bay was exercise, so I continued to do all I could to stay on top of it. I was on my second NDIS plan and had the ability to advocate for my support workers and find the appropriate people that suited my personality. I felt I had gained more confidence at this stage of my life to know who and what was good for me. I believe this was due to having more self-awareness through my 12-step Al-Anon program and my faith and trust in God.

Before my HSP diagnosis, I had decades of disbelief and judgement from some people and medical professionals because I had hemifacial dystonia, and I will always be grateful to a small group of Australians I found on an overseas group that I could relate to. Over time a few of the members started an Australian Dystonia Support Group. This group of amazing people became my friends as we helped each other through each day. Once I was diagnosed with a rare genetic progressing disease, I knew I needed to gain awareness and understanding into HSP. I was now trying to live and cope with two very challenging neurological disorders and there wasn't much awareness or understanding of either of them.

Hereditary Spastic Paraplegia (HSP) is a broad group of inherited, degenerative disorders characterised by impaired walking due to spasticity and weakness of the legs. The primary features of HSP are spasticity and weakness, with the proportions varying from individual to individual. Symptoms generally worsen over time, though by how much and how fast is highly variable. Diagnosis is primarily by clinical neurological examination and testing, as there are similarities with a number of other disorders. Genetic testing for HSP is now widely available. The detection rate of HSP mutations is in the 50 – 60% range with state-of-the-art next-generation whole exome sequencing.

HSP was first mentioned in 1876 by Adolph Seeligmüller, a German neurologist, who described a family of four affected children with spasticity. Further cases were described in 1883 by Adolph Strümpell, a German neurologist. Those cases were described more extensively in 1888 by Maurice Lorrain, a French physician. Due to their contribution in describing the disease, it is still named Strümpell-Lorrain disease in French-speaking countries. The term "hereditary spastic paraplegia" was coined by Anita Harding in 1983.

Even though I was an admin, and I loved working and supporting and organising support gatherings in the HSP Australian Support Group, I was also frustrated that there was no understanding, awareness, cure, or government funding. I often wondered that if there was a high profile identity with HSP, this disease would be given more recognition and status. Our Australian HSP Support Group was growing; we now had over 300 members and we knew there were at least 1800 people within Australia living with HSP. I was very passionate about trying to find them because with this disease you definitely needed a sense of belonging in order to live with the challenges. Our HSP support group had become like family to us all. I had the privilege of meeting many of the members, and they were the biggest blessing to me as we shared our lives from the bottom of our hearts. I was often enjoying a friendly chat over the phone. It was quite remarkable how close we had become.

We were going into our fourth year by this stage and I found managing the group satisfying but also time consuming. I felt pleased to find a few members who were willing to arrange a support gathering for their location in Australia. I also had a couple of great admins helping me run this friendly support group.

At this stage of my life, even though Greg and I were positive and enthusiastic, we wondered where this restrictive lifestyle was leading us. Greg continued to support and help me in any way he could. I was busy caring for my mother and/or attending NDIS appointments with the help of a support worker, while Greg continued to keep the home fires burning.

Our dog Jesse was three when my mother had the first stroke, and now he was almost ten, and in the early stages of heart failure. He had also gone deaf, so it had become easier and safer for Greg to stay home and walk him in his own environment. We had to make a lot of adjustments to all areas of our lives and we were both grateful for our faith in God because we knew this life was temporary and we often called our lifestyle the "New Normal". I relied on the prayer in Psalm 90:12—"Teach us to number our days, that we may gain a heart of wisdom", because I knew life was fragile and precious.

Susan Nicholson

Epilogue
SUSAN'S STORY CONTINUES....

Chapter 26
Celebrations and Struggles

Chris was turning 40 in December of 2019 and I was wanting to finish my memoir for him for his birthday. As well as being traumatised by the horrendous suffering my mother was enduring, having a rare, progressing, genetic disease meant I felt an urgency to write my own story. When I was feeding and caring for my mother at the nursing home, I could see so many beautiful souls passing away, with their own unique stories left untold. Just in case there were complications with my own health, I was determined to leave my story as a legacy to both my children.

Chris arranged for our family to go up to Sydney for Christmas and the celebration of his big 40th birthday! I arranged for some amazing friends to feed and care for my mother while we were away for the five days. Leaving my beloved mother was always emotionally traumatic for me, but in this case, I had no choice but to trust that the friends caring for my mother would do an amazing job. Able to communicate to my mother that I would be away for only five days, tears welled up in her eyes as she showed her understanding by nodding an acceptance of "yes". My heart always broke having to leave her, and this time was no exception.

I was so excited to finally give *Life, Loss and Love* to both Chris and Matthew, as I had poured my heart and soul into the pages of this memoir to them. Leaving it with them, I was keen for them to read it and give their opinion. I was delighted when they both came back and said they loved the read, expressing that there were so many raw emotions and truths in the content that they had been unaware of. My anxiety about self-publishing it was soothed when Matthew encouraged me by saying "The people who don't have a voice never get criticised, but they never reach their full potential!" This was enough for me to keep pushing on to publish my memoir, making it available for anyone who would be happy to pick it up and read it!

Chris's 40th birthday celebration was a fabulous time away in Sydney, and it was wonderful to be around both my children, their wives and my three little grandchildren, as well as my sister Maree and her husband. We were treated to an amazing day, driving around in a bus, and enjoying a delicious Italian meal all together, followed by a family day on Bondi Beach. Sadly, Maree and I were unable to join everyone at the beach. At the stage we were at with the progression of Hereditary Spastic Paraplegia, we were prevented from walking unaided and trying to walk in sand would be impossible. Chris and Linda had thought of everything and arranged for us to be at a delightful restaurant/club *Icebergs*, which had the most magical view of the sea. We felt so grateful to be loved and for our needs to be accommodated, in amongst all the logistics that went into catering for the needs of my little grandchildren and for Maree's and my disability.

I came home with renewed strength and feeling more relaxed to take on the intensive care my beautiful mother required! The amazing support I received from friends still available to help me, and the much-needed breaks on the days Maria or Rupsa could be feeding my mother, gave me such peace of mind! I had developed a beautiful relationship with one of my NDIS support workers, Manar, who came with me every time I was in with my mother. I felt as though I had struck gold, because Manar could intuitively see what my mother and I needed for help and support before I did! She was fast on her feet and could help me in so many ways! For example, while I was feeding my mother, Manar was able to spoon fluids into her mouth, because some days Mum could not remember to swallow. At this stage, my mother's cognition was not so good, but she was still very hungry and thirsty. After her lunch, we enjoyed playing uplifting sweet music to her, giving her a beautiful warm towel wash, and moisturising her face and hands. Mum looked so happy and contented after she was nice and full, and often would love just relaxing back in her bed chair and having a well-rested sleep. I felt so uplifted and secure, knowing I was leaving my mother very content. At this stage of her life, she was now in a place of acceptance and showed no signs of her earlier aggressive behaviour. Now that Manar was with me every time I went in, I felt so much happier. The whole experience for Mum and I was so much more enjoyable!

My precious mother was still alive and fighting the good fight! She was so determined and unwilling to give up, and I admired her for this quality of strength and resilience. I knew she had passed this character trait on to me because I was also incredibly determined! During the years of looking after her, especially after the first stroke, Mum always used to scream at me that she was not as strong as me when I was pushing her to keep going. I beg to differ because my mother is the strongest and most determined person I have ever known!

Greg and I had planned and booked a five-week round Australia cruise, never thinking when we did the booking that my mother would still be with us. I was receiving emails saying I had to pay the balance of the cruise in a matter of days and was experiencing severe anxiety at the thought of leaving my mother for a whole five weeks. I knew how difficult she was to feed. It used to take me hours, and although my sister, Maria and Rupsa would be there to feed and care for my mother, I just could not get any peace about leaving her for so long! She fed and behaved much better for me. I could not get my head around how on earth I was supposed to enjoy myself on the cruise. I just could not imagine wining and dining and going-to concerts, knowing my mother needed me so much. I was really struggling also because this was a trip we had planned as part of celebrating Greg's 70th birthday. It did not seem fair to not put my kind, caring and steadfast husband first for a change! After all, I could only give my mother this sort of time and energy because Greg was keeping our home functioning, and he deserved this wonderful time away from all the pressures of our daily lives.

I was also excited because I was going to be in Perth, and I would finally be able to meet all our members from our Hereditary Spastic Paraplegia Australian Support Group that I had founded in 2016. Our group was growing bigger by the day, and they were all excited to meet me. A large gathering was being planned, so I could meet as many members as I could while I was over in their part of Australia! Our friendships were growing as we all shared our ongoing struggles and challenges. HSP is an exceedingly difficult progressing disease to live with, and sharing our daily lives with each other was one of the ways we all kept going. We could also have a laugh at ourselves and with each other, which was so uplifting. I had planned this trip for so long and did not want to let anyone down, but my stomach was flipping all the time. I knew I had to give over a lot of money and having a mother in a nursing facility meant I was unable to receive any travel insurance. I prayed and took everything to God and I still had no peace! I had to ask myself: "If I was away for two weeks and I received news that my mother wasn't doing well, could I remain on the cruise and just enjoy it!" I did not have to think about it—the answer was

NO! I knew Greg would be fine, but I would be a total mess! So, once I had my answer, I was able to break it to Greg gently that we would have to cancel his long-awaited 70th birthday cruise in favour of me being with my beloved mother!

To honour Greg for being the wonderful husband he was to me, I was still wanting to celebrate his big 70th birthday. I was so excited when I was able to find an Italian restaurant willing to open for us to have an exclusive function for our family and friends! This meant we had the restaurant to ourselves. I invited all of Greg's siblings and his children and grandchildren. They all had to travel to be with him on his special day and it was a mighty effort getting almost everyone to come and be available on the same day! I invited some very special and loyal friends who had supported both Greg and me in our marriage and our ongoing health issues. Both Chris and Matthew, their wives and their children were all present.

We were able to set up an Art and Craft table for the seven little children who would be attending. I ordered a beautiful array of balloons and party bags so they could take them home and feel special, even though it was a celebration of 70 years well lived for Greg! We had a divine cake made, full of musical instruments, because Greg was a musician and songwriter. It was truly a birthday that we will all remember forever, because the unconditional love, acceptance and amazing speeches said it ALL!

Chapter 27
A Pandemic Emerges

My HSP continued to progress, and I was now using a scooter to walk our little King Charles Cavalier, Jesse. Poor Jesse was in chronic heart failure and was unable to walk far without getting very breathless, so we had bought a pet stroller for him that was just perfect for his walks. I enjoyed it so much more because I could look up and enjoy the beautiful ponds and wildlife where we lived. Greg was an amazing support to me, always making sure my mobility scooter was charged up ready for any adventure/outing we needed to go on!

We were a bit of a sight, but we all felt grateful we could still enjoy our lives and we found ways around everything we did! We had a wonderful friend Wendy who could clearly see we needed a little more support, so she used to give us some respite from the ongoing demands in medicating and getting Jesse out and about. On some occasions Wendy had Jesse stay with her up to five nights, so that gave both me and Greg a little break!

Life was quite difficult for me by now and I was using a walker inside our home to keep me from having a fall. I was doing a lot of wall surfing, just holding onto anything and everything to keep myself upright and safe! My grandchildren Behati, Leo and Chelsea were all growing up, and we had playdates any time we could. Chelsea was now over three years of age and I could have her more often for quality playdates on her own! We even found innovative ways to give Behati, who was now seven, and Leo, five, playtimes full of adventure and fun. Despite my physical limitations, we were giving them fabulous memories. My wonderful support worker Manar and I were able to take them on outings, because she could anticipate my needs and help keep us all safe!

It was all so priceless because the grandchildren loved their time with us, and I was very creative, making everything we did FUN! I even hired a Maxi Taxi and we were all picked up and taken out together, singing along as we went. I loved the way my grandchildren enjoyed hitching a ride on my walker. It made my heart skip a beat with pure delight to be having a relationship with my precious grandchildren that they would always remember!

Early one morning, I was getting ready to go in to feed and care for my mother, when my youngest son Matthew rang me. He was speaking quite fast and seemed to be very serious about taking me out with him to stock up on a few supplies of food and other items, which was not like him. Matthew, having done a double Economics degree, mentioned a serious deadly virus that he had been watching for quite some time, and he seemed extremely concerned for my safety and wellness. This was the first time I had heard of this virus, and I did not want to leave my mother, who needed intensive care, knowing that she would not get fed properly, if at all, if I were not there to do this for her.

I had seen enough of the aged care system to realise nothing could be trusted or relied upon, especially with the state of health my mother was in! She was at the mercy of the nursing home for absolutely everything, and they had a policy that if her eyes were closed or she did not understand, that meant she did not require a drink or a meal. I did not take Matthew seriously and did not want to leave my mother, even for a day, because I knew she would be neglected! I went in with Manar and we did all the essential requirements for my mother, not really thinking of what my son Matthew had been trying to tell me!

Listening to the news later that night I learned about a coronavirus—known as COVID-19—that was coming out of China, with many people overseas becoming infected. At this stage, I did not realise how serious this disease was. All our lives— and the whole world—were about to change dramatically!

The word "lockdown" was to become a harsh reality for us. One day in mid-March 2020, I was contacted urgently by Maria. She had been in feeding my mother when she was informed that the nursing home was going into lockdown. Upon hearing this devastating news, both my sister and I were extremely distressed, and we organised to visit our mother to explain to her what was happening. My mother appreciated truth, and even though she was so unwell I knew to give her all the facts that I had because she did not suffer fools gladly! I explained to her that there was a very contagious virus and because of this, the nursing home did not want any visitors—including family—coming in from the outside. I reassured Mum that she would be alright, and I told her that she had to eat and drink anything she was offered. In tears, and with limited understanding, she comprehended what I was saying, because she knew all about the Spanish Flu of 1918 (one of the deadliest pandemics in history).

I was so distressed I felt as though I would fall to pieces, and I could not resist saying to the nursing home workers that my mother was not going to die from this coronavirus, but from neglect! I felt sick to my stomach knowing I—and anyone else— was prohibited from getting in to help my mother. I was desperate to link up with her via Zoom so I could see and talk to her regularly, but it was just awful trying to communicate with my beloved mother. In the beginning, Mum could see me, and she appeared bright and we could understand each other (even though she was nonverbal). But the experience was horrendous for us both, and we shed countless tears.

Matthew and Krystal had decided to take Behati and Leo out of school, asserting that if the Prime Minister could not make the tough decision, then they would! The situation was escalating so quickly, and the news reports kept changing moment by moment. Because I knew so little about the virus, I was beside myself with worry and felt as though I was barely keeping my head above water. So much of our lives were being disrupted and everything appeared to be in total disarray.

Greg and I were trying to get our shopping done, and this was difficult because I needed my scooter to get around quickly. People were panic buying, and there was nothing left on the shelves, having been completely cleaned out by healthy able-bodied people. Suddenly, I was prevented from being close to my grandchildren and instead was only allowed to speak with them at a distance from our car. The whole situation felt so strange, so scary, and extremely traumatic. Our world was changing so quickly!

Our Prime Minister announced that state borders were all locking down, and we were advised not to travel. We were required to stay at home, only going out for essential things such as groceries, or travelling to and from work. We had to wash and sanitise our hands regularly, and not put them near our face. There was a myriad of instructions coming through the air waves almost constantly. It was such a strange way we were all living, but we were doing all we were told to try and prevent the spread of COVID-19. I was watching what was happening overseas, where the loss of life was heartbreaking, but we seemed to be in a good position compared to some other countries such as Italy and the United Kingdom.

My beloved mother was hanging in there, but I was feeling quite sick because I could not get in to see her. Over Zoom I could see she was looking unkempt and was going downhill fast, and I was inconsolable in my grief and distress. Over a period of time, she seemed to hear my voice, yet was unable to find me on the screen. I felt so helpless and powerless! All the years I had advocated for her—moving her to five different nursing facilities and helping her through so many hospital admissions and rehabilitations—felt as though it was all going to waste, because I had promised her while ever the good Lord gave me breath, I would never leave her nor forsake her.

Both Chris and Matthew had seen me giving care to my mother over the past seven years, and they were extremely concerned about the toll the situation was taking on my health and wellbeing. In between all of this, I was trying to be available for my three beautiful grandchildren, but with HSP progressing, Greg having memory issues and our little Jesse in heart failure, I felt overwhelmed! I kept trying to be grateful for what we still had left, but it was a major concern that the coronavirus was so insidious, with so little known about it at this stage.

Greg and I took the advice to stay at home seriously, and we did not go out much during this time. I would read or watch a good movie to divert my mind. Over Zoom, we were able to see Chris, Matthew, and their families, and it was so good to have a laugh and hook up with each other all together. I continued to work hard in our Hereditary Spastic Paraplegia Australian support group, and to stay connected and provide a sense of belonging, we decided to have three weekly chat rooms going. It was wonderful and uplifting to be able to see each other and talk about what was happening in our daily lives and our ongoing challenges.

As new COVID-19 cases spread, we saw international and domestic air flights discontinued. We had cruise ships stranded at sea with no Australian states willing to allow their passengers entry. I found it hard to believe that, had we taken that cruise around Australia for those five weeks (departing in February 2020), we would have been caught up in the situation, with the possibility of contracting the coronavirus ourselves. I could see God's hand at work in this situation because I always prayed for His will for our lives, and if I had no peace in a decision, I took it to mean God did not want us to pursue it. I had to rely totally on my strong faith at this stage of my life, because there was so much devastation and loss everywhere I turned!

Chapter 28
Grief Beyond Belief

It was April 21, and I was at home. Within a matter of a few hours, I had received three text messages from three friends, saying our Prime Minister was allowing visitors into nursing homes. I was quick to contact the nursing home and ask if I could come in to see my mother, with the response that visitors were not allowed. I decided to ring one of the only carers who would tell me the truth, and when I asked her about my mother, she said she had not eaten or had anything to drink that day and seemed to have lost that fight in her.

I emailed, texted and rang the Manager of the facility, and eventually she said if my mother was unwell then I could come in! I was delighted but also quite frightened because I had to wear a mask, gloves, and gown. Because of my mobility they allowed Greg to come in with me. I thought I would see my mother out in her bed chair and dressed, but to my shock and horror she was in bed, looking absolutely dreadful, and labouring to breathe! Immediately, I asked for her doctor to come in. Apparently, she had been in that state all day, yet at no stage was I rung to say she was so sick!

By now it was 4.00 pm, and my mother knew I was there as soon as she heard my voice; she could hear everything even though her eyes were hardly open. Silent tears streamed down her face, and she looked cold and unkempt, wearing only a threadbare, blue nightie. It was an utterly gut-wrenching scene. To make matters worse, the few carers wanted nothing to do with us—nor we with them—because everyone was terrified of catching the coronavirus.

I comforted my mother, wiping her beautiful face, neck, and body with a warm towel to help her feel better. I talked to her, trying to stay strong to keep her calm, even though I felt so heartbroken within to find her in this disgraceful state. I believed the three messages I received were from God, because I was able to advocate to get in to see my mother and assess the situation for myself! Waiting for the doctor to come in felt like forever, and when he finally did attend, he failed to examine her. I wanted him to organise a drip with fluids to be put up. His response was that nursing homes do not do this, but I was free to take her to a hospital. I knew my mother would not survive a hospital admission. Besides this, it was a cold night and it felt criminal to take her out in the state she was in, not to mention that the risk of contracting the coronavirus was great enough in a nursing facility. Why then would I want to risk the greater possibility of my mother contracting the disease from a hospital? The doctor and a registered nurse kept closing the door to my mother's room, and I could not believe the pressure both were putting on me to just let her go. The doctor wanted to set up a morphine driver, to which I responded, "You just want me to kill my mother off!" By now, I was sobbing uncontrollably. The doctor kept asking me when was the last time my mother had eaten or had a drink, to which I replied "How would I know? I haven't been allowed in to feed her for the last five weeks!" Neither could the few staff who were around provide him with an answer, as I could tell they simply did not have a clue.

I was screaming, "You have to get her out of the struggle to breathe—urgently!", but the pressure was put on me to decide there and then what to do about the situation. With my head pounding, and feeling so alone with such an enormous decision to make, I rang both my sons and my sister. I had a call from Maria and Manar, and they could tell I was all alone in it all! Manar jumped in her car and drove across town, but because they only allowed one person in at a time, she was forbidden to come in. Maria wanted to come across and stay with me, but I was not in my right mind to even consider what she was saying. It was all a big blur!

Chris sent me a text saying he was coming over and I remember responding "I need you!" The doctor told me to tell all my family, so that is what I did. He changed his mind and offered a miniscule amount of morphine to make my mother comfortable, which seemed reasonable to me. It was now 7.30 pm, and my beloved mother was administered the small amount of morphine for comfort. My sister and her son came and spent some time with Mum. I wanted to discuss the next plan of action with my sister, but her son was content to say he was grateful that his Nan was at peace. Of course she was, because of the morphine administered just before they arrived!

I was still so distressed. Chris came in and had some quality time with me and his grandmother, and at no stage did I think my beloved mother would be dying. I stayed until midnight, watching the clock because our Jesse was overdue for his heart medication. Greg was unable to medicate the dog without me, and we lived a good 30 minutes' drive away, so I had to go home. With a massive headache from the stress I left, saying I would have my mobile on loud and to give me a call if my mother showed any signs of distress. I came home and got my clothes out, ready to be up early the next day and back in with my mother so we could weigh up the options and speak to the doctor. In hindsight, I really needed a female with me, and both Maria and Manar were so loving, kind and caring and would have stayed with me. I was exhausted and keen to have a few hours' sleep, get rid of the headache, and get back to my mother.

I was devastated when I received a phone call at 4.00 am to say my mother had passed away! I was in total shock, because the doctor had said we would discuss the next step in the morning. When I think about it, he was unable to get an answer as to whether my mother had any fluids on board. Even though she was given the tiniest amount of morphine, I believe it was enough to give comfort and my mother passed away! I will forever regret not staying the rest of the night, but with my head pounding, I was in no fit state to be there. Hindsight is a great teacher, and I should have taken something for the headache and gone back across with Maria or Manar. If I did not have HSP I could have driven back over, but I was struggling so badly and needed help!

I could not believe I had worked so hard to keep my mother so clean and well fed yet was unable to be with her when she passed from this life to the next! My beautiful mother had died alone, and it felt as though all the time, unconditional love, and energy I put into caring for her was wasted. The small dose of morphine that had been administered would have only lasted until 1.30 am, so there would have been no further pain relief to assist her. Goodness knows what distress my mother may have gone through before she took her final breath. Because she was not found by staff until 4.00 am, I will never know the full details—and the truth—of her passing. I felt it had ended really badly, and to this day, I still have not found any peace around how it all unfolded. I believe I was pressured to let my mother go without knowing—or being offered—the full facts of her situation.

Now it was time to start ringing family members to let them know Mum had passed away. I said I would ring my sister, but I was informed it was a policy of the nursing home that they would be the ones to do this! I sat up in bed distressed, shocked and in the deepest of grief, knowing I was prevented from going into the nursing home due to all the stringent Coronavirus rules. I also felt defeated, and wondered to myself what use going in would be.

I rang both Chris and Matthew and told them that their beloved grandmother had passed away. I had not heard from Maree and believed this was because she was distressed and trying to process it all! I was in so much grief and emotional pain and there was no one to talk to. I waited until around 7.00 am and put a post on Facebook that my mother had passed away! I was in two closed Facebook groups—a carers support group and a prayer group. It gave me comfort that I was able to write something and receive some response from people who knew the long and distressing battle I had been fighting over the seven years of caring for my beloved mother.

Due to the COVID-19 restrictions, only ten people were allowed at her funeral. This was undoubtedly the saddest time of my life. Aware of my distress, the funeral directors suggested it may help me emotionally if we had a viewing of my mother's body. I do not believe in going to view the body of someone who has passed away, because I know they are no longer there, and their soul has gone to heaven. However, in this case I felt it might at least ease my painful memory of my beloved mother's distress. Memories of how she knew exactly what was going on around her; and of how her bedroom door was closed several times while the doctor and registered nurse applied pressure on me to let her go!

A few family members and friends came to the viewing because they would not be allowed to come to the funeral. I was relieved to see that my beloved mother looked nice; well-kept and with her hair done. I was able to place an earlier version of *Life, Loss and Love* that I had been reading to her, into her arms in the coffin. That gave me some sort of peace, that I had written this book and she loved listening to it, nodding with agreement at the content. I was so proud I had written a book where she had become the hero of my memoirs.

I looked at the death certificate, and it was signed off that my mother had pneumonia. I thought how untrue that was! She died from neglect and dehydration; it was as simple as that! I was angry, but I had to get a hold of myself, and accept that she was finally away from her struggling body, and alive in heaven with Jesus! This was the only way I was going to cope and survive—by going back to my revelation that I had when I became a born-again Christian decades before! I needed to hold on to my faith and hope—that God knew everything and was still in control, because living in this world and the suffering made no sense to me at this stage of my life!

Chapter 29

Celebration of My Mother's Life!

The faithful priest who had walked with me in my suffering, loss and struggles all those decades before, and who had been a wonderful witness to me, helped us organise my beloved mother's funeral. He was wonderful to us, and it gave me so much more comfort to have him helping us all and officiating. It felt so good to be able to talk about Mum's life and who she really was. Greg and I, Maree and her husband Laurie arranged a lovely celebration of Mum's life, including Greg's song "Don't let your hearts be troubled", inspired by the words of Jesus in *The Book of John,* Chapter 14, in the Bible.

Even though it felt sad to have only ten people attend my mother's funeral, it was also somewhat of a relief for me, as my state of mind was not good. I felt extremely loved and cared for by so many people, as so many cards, flowers, phone calls, social media and text messages were flooding into our home. The beautiful fragrance of all the flowers was giving our home the sweetest scent that made me feel that Mum was around me in spirit.

My mother liked only the best and took great notice if the quality was not the real thing, so we picked a beautiful solid wood coffin. I worked on the words I wanted to say about my mother and the life she had led. She was a real character and she loved people. Rather than having only ten people attending, she would have wanted an enormous celebration of her life! I decided we needed a video of the funeral so we could share it with close family and friends, but I did not feel strong enough to have the service screened live. Due to the COVID-19 restrictions, the ten people allowed were Greg and me, Chris and Linda, Matthew and Krystal, Maree and Laurie and their son and his partner.

On the actual day of the funeral, I felt emotionally stronger and I was determined to do Mum proud, because that is what she would have wanted! I felt quite lost and lonely as we left, because we were not allowed to get together afterwards, so Greg and I went home by ourselves. It was such a strange, weird feeling, but so was everything at this stage of the lockdowns and restrictions. Later that night our family all hooked up with Zoom to talk to each other so we would have a feeling of belonging in our grief! I was so grateful that my friend Maria was willing to mind Behati and Leo, so Matthew and Krystal could come and relax for that short time of the celebration of Mum's life!

As the months went by, we decided to hold a memorial service for my mother. My sister Maree had organised a beautiful place to rest her ashes next to her loving partner Olek, as they had shared 28 years of their lives together! We decided as a family to say a few personal and private words about our relationship with our mother/grandmother. It was just beautiful because we could have a laugh at her funny ways, and each of us all had our own memories of her—it was so honest and transparent!

We booked a private room and had a beautiful lunch together where we could toast and celebrate her life. It was quite funny because my mother would not have approved of us treating ourselves to a fine dining lunch, because she was born during the Great Depression and would have thought, "What a waste of money!" I can still hear her saying, "Fools and their money are soon parted!" She was generous in so many ways, but not when it came to dining out.

So, both my sister and I agreed we had put in some horrendous and exhausting years, and we felt we needed to treat and be kind to ourselves for once! I had relief and comfort knowing my mother was finally away from her paralysed body. I also knew without a doubt she had just gone to her eternal reward and she would be waiting for me and all of those who die in Christ! I knew I was feeling exhausted and in deep grief, but I had hope that the pain would slowly subside, and I could continue on, living life with a grateful heart!

Chapter 30

Life Goes On In a COVID-19 World

We were all living the best life we could under the restrictions of the coronavirus. Both Greg and I had planned to do some travel, but since my mother has passed away, we have not been able to leave the Australian Capital Territory where we live in Australia. We are in a high-risk category with COVID-19, so we must keep ourselves as safe as we can be, living a quiet life in our comfortable home with Jesse. We undertake little outings to break the monotony, but we are hoping we can receive a vaccination that may give us a little more freedom to travel within Australia. Every day is different and our state borders close and open depending on the infection rates and community transmissions of COVID-19.

Living with HSP is still my biggest ongoing challenge. However, living in the grip of a pandemic has dramatically changed the way we live and go about our business. We are so grateful to be living in Australia compared to so many other countries that have had so much loss of innocent life to this deadly virus. We have our family and friends around us, and everyone is well. We are dealing with this strange new way of living.

I believe the biggest outcome of this pandemic has been the realisation of how much we took our freedom and way of life for granted. The lessons we have learned have been many—for example, having resilience and courage in the face of adversity as moment-to-moment the coronavirus pandemic sets the new rules around how we live our lives. We have learned to be grateful for the simple things in life—especially family and friends—and to treasure the moments spent together. A telephone call or a visit from a friend, looking out for your neighbour, and reaching out to your fellow man, are also the simple things in life which are the most important.

I continue to listen and pay attention to what is happening in every country around the world as it adapts to the ravages of the COVID-19 pandemic. The devastation and loss of life is something that has affected me deeply. Life is something which is precious and fragile, and this has never been more evident to me than at this present time. With no immediate end in sight, I continue to pray for all the people who are fighting this pandemic every day!

It is my hope that reading my memoir has also given you, dear reader, the realisation that life, though full of struggle and loss, can also be full of joy and love. As we come to terms with the realisation that our world has forever been changed because of the pandemic, let us look for the little things in life that bring us joy. Let us appreciate the beauty that is still in this world—that no pandemic can ever take away.

And, just like my beloved mother, who clung to life with grit and determination under horrific circumstances, let us celebrate the tenacity of the human spirit and the endurance to run the race of life well—to the very end. Only God knows when our race will be finished, and when this gift of life that He has given us will come to an end. So, let us appreciate this precious gift for everything it is worth, and let us decide to squeeze every single drop of life out of it that we can.

Acknowledgements

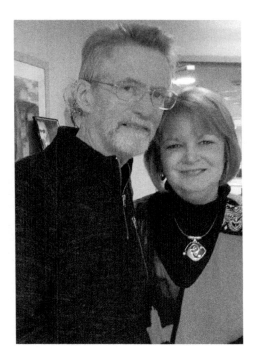

An enormous thank you to my steadfast and patient husband Greg. Without his nonstop, tireless help, this book would not exist. He believed in me when I wasn't sure I believed in myself. His love is more precious than gold. He had faith in me and sustained me when I thought I couldn't go on.

***

To Meredith Swift who encouraged me to follow the desires of my heart and write my story and my truth. I will always have so much gratitude and appreciation.

Please Leave a Review

I would like to take the time to thank everyone who has read my memoir and who have taken the time to give me a review! It is the most humbling feeling that my story has inspired and helped others who have experienced loss.

Could you please leave a review on Amazon at https://www.amazon.com/dp/B088Q1YVSL and/or Goodreads to let me know what you think of my book. Each review is worth its weight in gold and I would be so grateful if you could do this.

If you would like to correspond with me, about any aspect of my story, please feel free to contact me at: suzmorandini@gmail.com.